AVOIDING MISCARRIAGE

everything you need to know to
feel more confident in pregnancy

SUSAN ROUSSELOT

Foreword by noted miscarriage specialist
Dr. Mary Stephenson, MD
Professor of Obstetrics and Gynecology

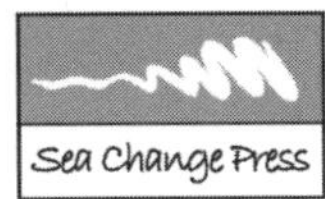

First printing.

ISBN 0-9774933-1-8.

Library of Congress Control Number: 2005910063.

Design, photographs and illustrations:

Cover design by Peta Nugent.

Author photos by Daniel Rousselot, Paris: www.daniel-rousselot.net.

Front cover photos licensed from Getty Images.

Illustration by Ian Faulkner: www.ianfaulknerillustrator.com.

Visit this book's website at www.avoidingmiscarriage.com for additional information, support, and resources.

acknowledgements

I owe a debt of gratitude to all those people who helped make this book possible

To the women who shared their personal experiences of loss – your courage fuelled my determination to write this book. Special thanks to those who allowed their stories to be included, and who provided indispensable insights in shaping the book: Melinda Conrad, Laura Martin Medina, Collette Harkins, Jill Perrin, Michelle Blaine, Debbie Zerbst, Sara Landa, Michele Corin, Jennifer Caldwell, Helen Fraser, and Tiffany Foster, as well as Catherine, Popi, and Elizabeth, who prefer to remain anonymous.

To Dr. Mary Stephenson, Dr. Patrick Riley, Dr. Daniel Abbott, and Dr. Laura Riley for their valuable input on this project.

To researchers, doctors, and healthcare professionals working to reduce miscarriage and improve women's reproductive outlook – your work is greatly appreciated.

To Diane Zoi, Betsy Golden, Karen Ivey, Jessica Hollander, Lisa Martin, and James Leibert for vital strategic, editorial, logistical, and moral support on this book and others.

And finally, to my husband and children, for their unfailingly generous encouragement and sense of humor. Without them, this book simply would not exist.

about the author

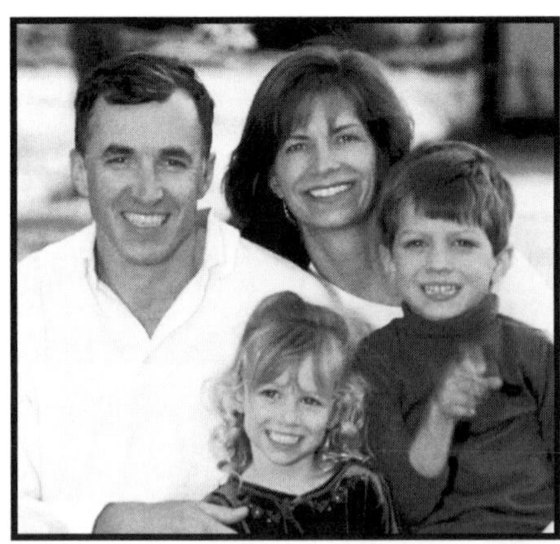

Susan Rousselot draws on both training and personal experience to write this empowering and informative book. With degrees from Wellesley and MIT, and experience as a medical researcher, she has tracked down and deciphered the most solid, up-to-date medical information. Yet she covers the subject with a clarity that comes from being an accomplished author, and a compassion that comes from her own miscarriages; she knows firsthand the many difficult issues that pregnancy loss can trigger, and how hard it can be to get answers. She translates complex medical research into clear language and useful insights, and presents it all with sensitivity and optimism. Finally, she encourages readers by her own example, because although she knew nothing about miscarriage when it struck her, she resolved to take an informed, positive role in her own healthcare, and believes her two children are the direct result.

By sharing her experience and research, Susan hopes to help other women avoid miscarriage.

dedication

To Jean-Baptiste, Roland and Jacqueline

who make everything seem possible.

A note from the author

This book is intended to help you decipher the medical advice you may get, and better understand your options. It is not intended to replace medical consultation.

As your situation is unique, and because medical information can change rapidly, I strongly encourage you to discuss all health matters, questions, and concerns with your physician before embarking on any diagnostic or treatment strategies.

A disclaimer from the legal department

table of contents

"Destiny is no matter of chance.

It is a matter of choice.

It is not a thing to be waited for,

It is a thing to be achieved."

(William Jennings Bryan; 1860-1925)

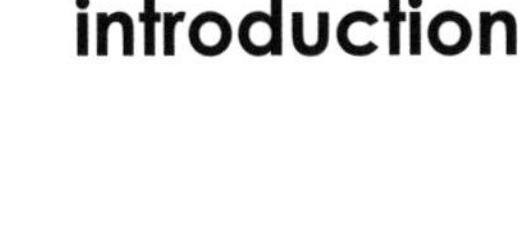

introduction

foreword

As Director of the Recurrent Pregnancy Loss Program, I see many couples suffering the devastation of pregnancy loss. While the grief of loss is itself a heavy burden to bear, there are often a number of other upsetting issues that miscarriage raises. Many couples feel confused and guilty about pregnancy loss, and frustrated or powerless in their search for answers.

Miscarriage is one of the most common reasons that healthy women require medical attention. Yet despite it being so terribly prevalent, miscarriage can also be terribly isolating. The whole experience can be highly stressful and unbalancing.

For anyone concerned about miscarriage, it is important to get answers and support. My colleagues and I strive to provide this by working with couples to give them as many answers as possible, and by continuing to research miscarriage causes and treatments. In addition to our goals of providing the information and assistance patients need to move forward more confidently, our ultimate goal is for couples to avoid miscarriage.

Author Susan Rousselot has the very same goals, and she succeeds admirably in this book. Presented in a supportive and encouraging way, *Avoiding Miscarriage* provides comprehensive, up-to-date information addressing the many questions that couples may have about miscarriage. It also helps women look at the specifics of their own situation, and evaluate their own options.

Through this book, women can get a thorough understanding of the subject of miscarriage, reflect on their own areas of increased risk, and clarify how vigorously they want to pursue answers. With these insights they can work more effectively with their doctors to get the healthcare they want, and focus on issues or concerns of particular relevance to them.

I recommend this book for both patients and medical professionals alike. With its meticulous research, useful information, and poignant insights, there is much for anyone to learn here.

This book encourages women to take an informed role in their own healthcare, which is an idea that I thoroughly support. In my experience, women who do so reap a double benefit: not only is it a psychologically positive, healthy thing to do, but it often brings the goal of successful pregnancy that much closer.

If you are concerned about your own risk of miscarriage, the road you are on can be difficult and fraught with anxiety. This book is written to help make your road to success shorter and easier.

By picking up this book you have already taken a constructive step toward your future, and I wish you every success in creating the happy, healthy family that you want.

Mary Stephenson, MD, MSc

Professor of Obstetrics / Gynecology
Director, Recurrent Pregnancy Loss Program
The University of Chicago Hospitals

about this book

Why I wrote this book

Although I now have two lovely children, achieving motherhood was a real challenge. I had six miscarriages, and wherever I looked, answers were too hard to find. My doctor was unhelpful, books didn't tell me anything about my own situation, and the Internet was bewildering.

After exhaustive research I found that all I needed was low-dose aspirin which I could buy at the corner store. Had this book existed when I needed it, I would have avoided several miscarriages.

While experiencing recurrent miscarriage as I did is very rare, having one miscarriage is quite common. Despite the fact that miscarriage strikes nearly one in every five pregnancies, it is still a subject cloaked in mystery and fear. There is much comfort to be gained from clearing away the confusion and getting solid answers.

I wrote this book so that other women don't have to go through what I did – so they can feel more confident in pregnancy, have more effective relationships with their doctors, and ultimately avoid miscarriage.

Who this book is for

This book is for any woman who wonders what she can do to reduce her chance of miscarriage and create a better future. It is written for:

Women who have never been pregnant. If you want to find out about the conditions that cause miscarriage, and whether you could be at increased risk for any of them, then this book is for you.

Women who want to make informed decisions about delaying childbearing. It can be very difficult to find the information you need to understand how age affects your risk profile. This book presents the facts and discussion you need to make informed decisions.

Women who have miscarried. With its targeted questionnaires and miscarriage evaluation flowcharts, this book can help you find specific answers and clarify the way forward.

Women who want to take charge of their reproductive healthcare. Whether it is forging a partnership with your doctor or creating an effective, easy-to-use action plan, this book is designed to help you achieve the balance and results you want.

About the cases, research, and numbers

The case studies

There are several case studies included in this book, recounting the personal experiences of real women. These women were not recruited from any group, nor were they screened for what they had to say. To find them I simply sent an e-mail to close friends, asking if they, or one of their own close friends, had a story of miscarriage they were willing to share.

These are the stories of family, friends, colleagues, and people that surround us in daily life; they include those of my sister, a childhood friend, a colleague, and my daughter's teacher, among others. It amazed me that so many people in my close circle had been through such experiences – most had never mentioned them before. Such silence is a common, painful feature of miscarriage.

The research

In researching this book I read hundreds of medical reports, articles, and books, and sought clarification and further information from several medical professionals.

While the Internet and the popular press can be very useful sources, they can also be inaccurate, misleading, or incomplete, as they are not subject to the same stringent guidelines, controls and reviews as reputable medical journals.

On the other hand, information from medical journals, medical research centers and well-researched books is more reliable, but often technical or hard to understand.

In this book I have tried to combine the best of both worlds by using sound medical data, but explaining it like a friend.

The numbers

Unfortunately, miscarriage is a field in which numbers are often lacking or conflicting. But I know how useful it is to have solid figures, so on the basis of all my research, I have included those that seemed the most consistent, reliable and informative.

About gender

Throughout this book I refer to doctors in the masculine. This is for nothing more than practical typesetting reasons, as "he" and "his" are shorter than "he or she" and "his or hers." There are both male and female doctors doing excellent work in the field of miscarriage.

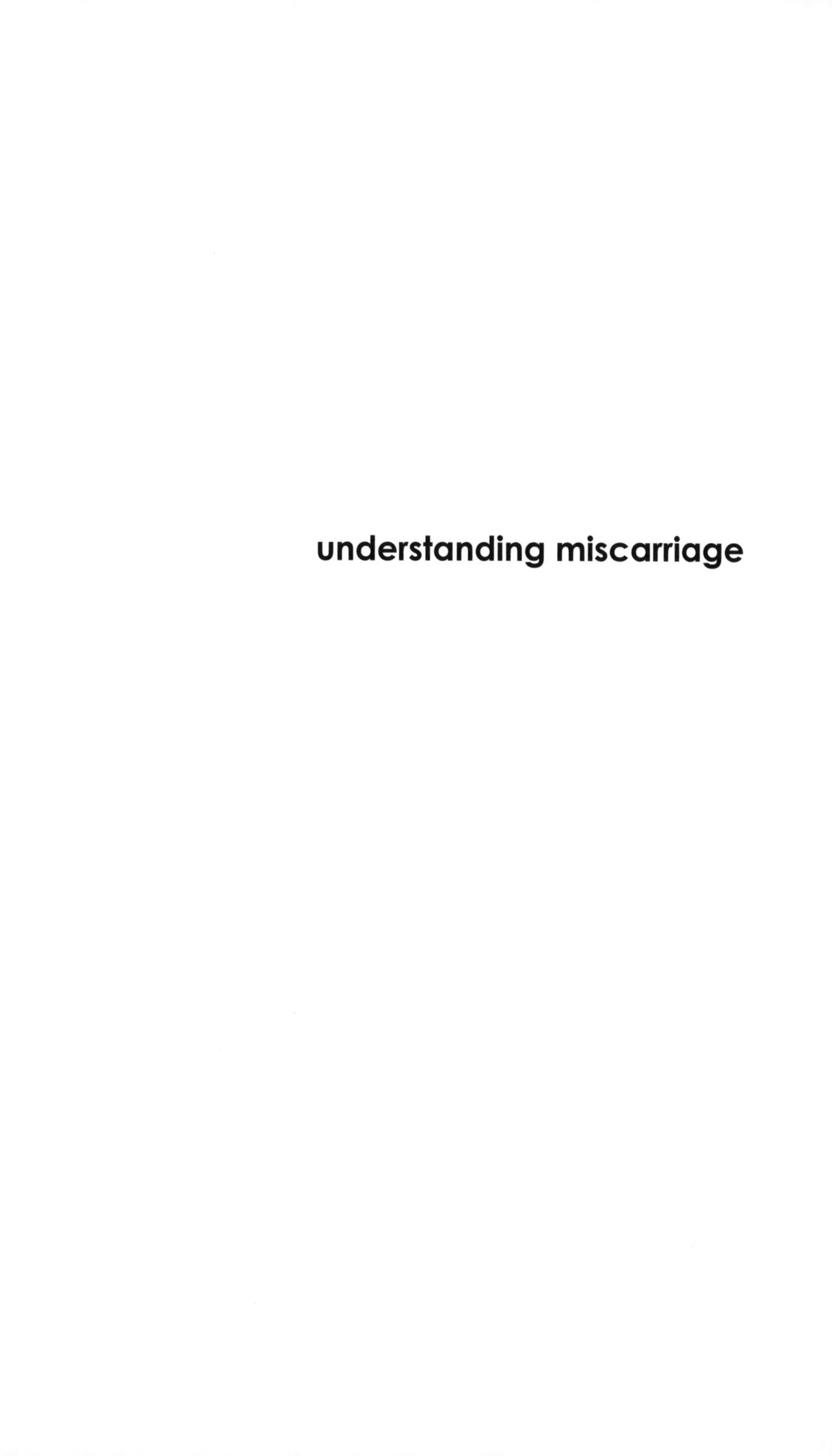

understanding miscarriage

miscarriage explained

Melinda's story

We started trying to have kids when I was 33. After I went off the pill my cycle was very irregular, with six or seven weeks between periods. When we weren't pregnant after about six months, I consulted a fertility specialist, who immediately put me on Clomid. I felt as if suddenly the process was being dictated by a fertility specialist – it was like: "Try this, then move up to the next level; try that, then move up to the next level." I was on a conveyor belt going towards a goal I didn't want. It was his process, not something that was right for me. I had a sense that I shouldn't go down this path with nothing in my history to indicate that it was really warranted.

I hated Clomid, and had terrible side-effects, so went off it after a few months. We got pregnant right after.

I miscarried at seven or eight weeks. The miscarriage itself was physically painful, and I didn't know when it was appropriate to go to the hospital. I'll never forget pulling out all my pregnancy books to try to figure out how much bleeding meant I should go to the hospital, and whether or not I would need a D&C. I felt really alone. It was a very private thing, and I didn't want to share it, but I didn't want to be alone, either.

The hospital doctor was great. She told me, "You have no idea how many women have miscarriages – it's really, really, common." That made me feel much better. There was still that "Oh God, what's wrong with me? It's all my fault!" voice in my head, but I did feel better.

I found the loss extremely tough. I thought either you could have babies or you couldn't, and panicked that the miscarriage meant that I couldn't. I was surprised by how traumatic the experience was, and had no idea where to turn to for support.

After the miscarriage my cycle went back to how it was before – it was very irregular and I couldn't seem to get pregnant.

I confided in a good friend who told me about an MD who was achieving great success augmenting traditional Western medical care with natural therapies. Because that doctor is so in demand, I had to wait four months to get in to see her. But she was wonderful! She explained everything, gave me specific notes and a diagram of my ovulatory cycle, wrote down the vitamins I should be taking and why. She was amazing. I had a regular cycle in a month, and was pregnant in two.

After that there was no trouble at all; Sam was born happy and healthy. Afterwards I was back to my irregular cycle, but the same doctor had me regular again in no time, and I got pregnant shortly thereafter. I have just had my second son after an easy pregnancy.

I think there's way too much silence around the whole issue of miscarriage, which is a shame because so many people go through it. You don't realize how common it is – even among your own friends – because it's this unspeakable subject. It's like silent torture.

So when it happened to me, I thought I must have done something wrong. I couldn't understand why this had happened, and was desperate to find a reason, even if it was my fault.

Learning more about miscarriage made all the difference. When I found out how common it really is I felt this liberation. And when I realized that having a miscarriage meant my body could do the hard part, and that my chances of success the next time were really high, I felt this huge sense of relief, as if I could suddenly breathe again.

miscarriage explained

As Melinda discovered, the anxiety of miscarriage can be greatly reduced when fear and mystery are replaced by fact and clarity. This chapter is written with that goal in mind.

We've all heard the alarming news that miscarriage is more common than we thought, and that it is on the rise – it's even said that "most women can expect to have a miscarriage." Many of us have begun to pay more attention to reports and articles about miscarriage, hoping they might contain useful information or practical advice. Unfortunately, the more closely we look at the subject of miscarriage, the more confusing it can appear – each report seems to come up with different results, and each article seems to come to a different conclusion. Instead of painting a clearer picture of miscarriage, these conflicting viewpoints can make miscarriage seem even more mysterious and incomprehensible – it can be difficult to know what to believe. Worst of all, there is little or no information on what we can do to improve our odds of a healthy pregnancy.

Concerned women have some key questions about miscarriage that they want answered:

- What are the facts about miscarriage, and why does it happen?
- How common is it really, and is it on the rise?
- Is it true that "most women can expect to miscarry at least once"?
- Why do doctors seem reluctant to investigate miscarriage?
- Can I predict my own chance of miscarriage?
- And most importantly: Is there anything I can I do to avoid it?

The first four of these questions will be answered in this chapter, while the last two will be the focus of subsequent chapters.

Conception and early pregnancy

Before analyzing miscarriage, it is worth reviewing the reproductive process. A summary can be broken down into five steps:

Step 1: Fertilization. An ovary releases an egg into the fallopian tube, where it fuses with a sperm at conception. Unlike other cells, which all have 23 *paired* chromosomes (46 total), sperm cells have only 23 *unpaired* chromosomes. Egg cells have 46 chromosomes which separate into two sets of 23 unpaired chromosomes when a sperm enters the egg. One set pairs with the sperm's chromosomes, while the other is ejected. Only when egg and sperm correctly fuse do they create a full complement of 23 paired chromosomes. The chromosomes in this first cell are the blueprint for every other cell in the human body – 10 trillion of them by adulthood.

Step 2: Replication. Cell division begins about a day after fertilization, copying the 23 chromosome pairs formed at conception. The cell replicates its genetic material and then divides down the middle – making two identical cells where there was once only one. These two cells then replicate their genetic material, and divide again, making four cells from two. Those four cells then become eight, which become 16, and so on. The fertilized egg continues to travel down the fallopian tube toward the womb, even as it replicates its genetic material and divides.

Step 3: Implantation. About 7-10 days after fertilization the fertilized egg (called a "blastocyst" of about 128-256 cells) burrows into the lining of the womb. The placenta – at this stage a network of blood vessels – develops between it and the wall of the womb, supplying blood, oxygen and nutrients from the mother to the developing baby (now called an "embryo") via the umbilical cord.

Step 4: Growth. The embryo begins a phase of rapid growth and change. The cells begin to differentiate: first they form three distinct layers; later they will become every different structure and organ in the body. This explosive growth and development requires an ever-increasing supply of nourishment from the mother's body. By 8 weeks after conception (10 weeks' gestation) the baby is referred to as a "fetus."

Step 5: Birth. About 38 weeks after fertilization (40 weeks after the last menstrual period) the baby is ready to be born. The average baby will weigh 7½ pounds (3.4 kg) and be 20 inches (50 cms) long.

Why miscarriage happens

Generally, a pregnancy that combines a healthy embryo (steps 1-3, above) with a nourishing environment (steps 3 and 4, above) will progress to full term (birth). However, if there is a significant problem with either the embryo or the nourishment it receives in the womb, then the pregnancy is typically lost. If this loss occurs before 20 weeks gestation it is called a miscarriage; after that time it is termed a stillbirth.

Though the name "miscarriage" implies that a woman carried her pregnancy improperly (i.e. she mis-carried it), this is not at all the case. Miscarriage is caused by a variety of factors that interfere with one of the first four steps listed above. These factors – and what can be done to test for, treat, and counteract them – will be explained in detail.

The chance of having a miscarriage

Because miscarriage tends to be a highly personal and private experience, solid data on miscarriage can be difficult to get. Even worse, it can be hard to rely upon, as each study seems to present different numbers. This is not as confusing – or alarming – as it appears. The simple reason that miscarriage rates are difficult to compare from one report to the next is that the chance of miscarriage decreases dramatically during the first few days and weeks after fertilization. As illustrated on the chart below, miscarriage rates can vary widely if studies are looking at even slightly different timeframes.

As shown on the chart, the chance of a fertilized egg miscarrying at some point is about 75% – most fertilized eggs never even implant. However, once the egg *has* successfully implanted (still several days before the first period is due), the chance that it will miscarry before full term drops to about 30%.

Less than a week later – around the time the first period is due – the chance of miscarriage has dropped again. Pregnancies detected either by a missed period or a pregnancy test (whether at home or in a doctor's office) are called "confirmed pregnancies," and most experts agree that nearly 20% of these pregnancies end in miscarriage.

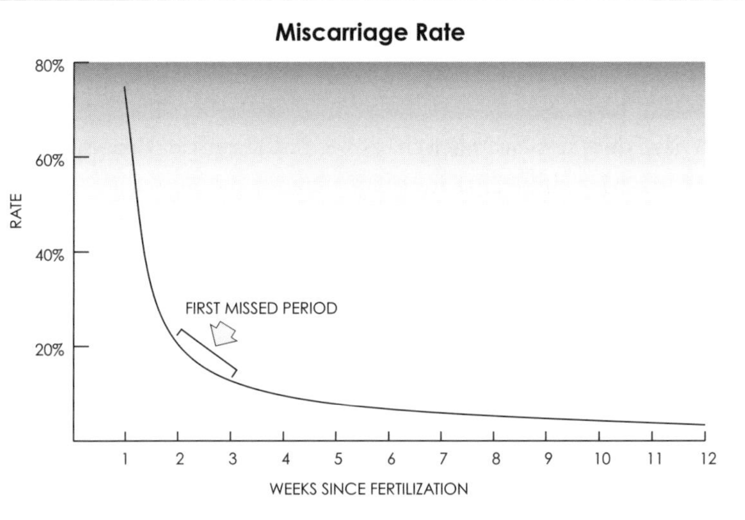

Illustrating the difficulties that can arise when comparing results of various studies, let us briefly consider a Danish study of more than a million pregnancies, which found only a 13.5% miscarriage rate. How could such a large study indicate a result so much lower than the 20% the experts believe? Probably because the Danish study was based on hospital data and women generally only require hospital attention if the pregnancy has progressed beyond the first few weeks. Women who miscarried in the first few days after their period was due may have called or consulted their doctors, but are unlikely to have checked into the hospital for treatment. These miscarriages – which are the most common – would therefore have gone unreported. Thus, while initially these two pieces of data seem to contradict each other, it is more likely that they are just looking at slightly different points on the curve shown in the chart above.

Consecutive miscarriages

For anyone who has experienced a miscarriage, the thought of having another is naturally a cause of great concern. Luckily, one miscarriage does not mean you are likely to have another.

A woman's chance of miscarriage does not increase perceptibly if she has already had one – it is still about 20%. (Unfortunately, having a miscarriage does not *lower* her chance of future miscarriage, either. It is not as if she has fulfilled her statistical quota and can now go on to four trouble-free pregnancies – she still has a one in five chance of miscarriage with each pregnancy.)

However, once a woman has had *two* miscarriages in a row, the likelihood of having a third rises to about 33%, or one in three. Three consecutive miscarriages indicate a woman's chance of miscarrying a fourth time is about 45%, or nearly one in two.

But consecutive miscarriages remain quite rare. Only about 5% of couples will have two miscarriages in a row, and only about 1% of couples – one in every 100 – will have three in a row.

The issue of maternal age

A miscarriage rate of 20% of confirmed pregnancies applies to the "average" woman (whoever she is). Of course, when evaluating our own chance of miscarriage, it is not enough to rely on population statistics. Each of us needs to understand and assess our own unique profile. And the most important factor in predicting miscarriage rate is maternal age (a woman's age at the time she becomes pregnant). But as with almost all conditions associated with miscarriage, many of the specific problems associated with advanced maternal age can be assessed and addressed in a number of ways.

Though it smacks of ageism, sexism and all sorts of "isms" seemingly designed to keep women barefoot, pregnant, and out of the boardroom, it has been irrefutably demonstrated that age plays a key role in a woman's chance of miscarriage. As shown below, miscarriage rates increase dramatically with maternal age, as the health and functioning of the reproductive system decline.

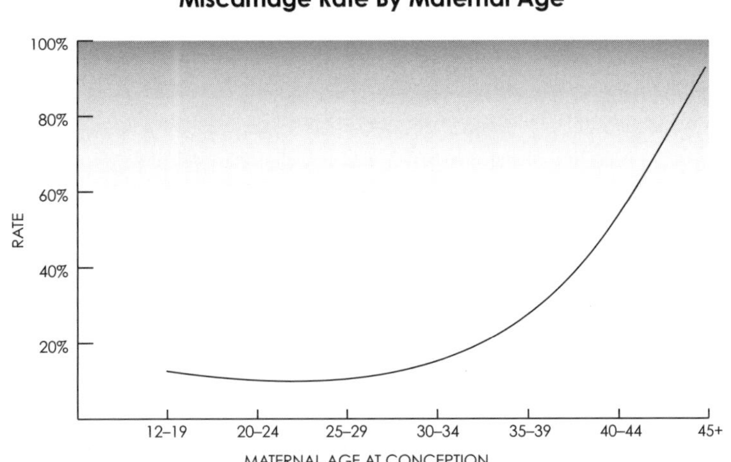

However, while "age" is often cited as the culprit, that can be misleading; it is how close a woman is to menopause that has a greater impact on cellular function and egg quality.

Unlike men, who produce sperm daily, women are born with ovaries stocked with eggs. Women have the most eggs (1-2 million) when they are still in their mother's womb. By the time women reach puberty and the onset of menstruation, the stock of eggs has declined markedly, and only about 300,000 remain. This reserve of eggs continues to drop, not because of ovulation, which uses only 400-500 eggs over a lifetime, but due to natural degeneration.

Before a woman is born, the eggs' process of replication and division stops mid-division. Each egg's division process remains arrested for the next 12-50 years, until it matures just prior to ovulation. At that time the process starts up again, and the first division is completed. One of the pair is ejected, leaving the other intact in the egg. A second division then begins, but stops once again at ovulation, restarting only if a sperm penetrates the egg. If a sperm does penetrate the egg, then at that point division resumes, producing two unpaired sets of maternal chromosomes. One set fuses with the sperm's chromosomes, creating a set of 23 paired chromosomes; the set of unpaired maternal chromosomes is ejected.

Needless to say, all this starting, stopping, dividing and ejecting is a risky way of working. And risk is only increased with 'age' (or, more accurately, proximity to menopause). This is because the cells surrounding the eggs play an important role in the eggs' healthy operation. These cells secrete hormones required to coordinate the eggs' proper functioning, and to support fertility. As the number of eggs decreases due to degeneration, hormone levels produced by the surrounding cells are also reduced. By the time only about 1,000 eggs remain, hormone levels are too low to maintain menstruation and menopause occurs.

The role of menopause

Lower egg reserves generate less hormone in the environment surrounding the egg, leading to more irregularities and malfunctions, and resulting in more genetic abnormalities. Thus, the closer a woman is to menopause (and the lower her egg reserve and surrounding hormone levels) the higher the likelihood of poor egg quality. This is demonstrated by the increased incidence of chromosomally abnormal births as women age:

	Frequency of a live birth with:	
Maternal age	**Down's**	**Any genetic abnormality**
25	1 in 1,400	1 in 476
30	1 in 800	1 in 385
35	1 in 380	1 in 164
40	1 in 110	1 in 51
45	1 in 30	1 in 15

Older eggs are associated with higher rates of genetic abnormality; so while only some of a 25-year old's eggs might be abnormal, by age 40 more than half of them might be. Older eggs are also more prone to errors in the fusion process with the sperm, with chromosomes breaking off or crossing over, resulting in genetic abnormality of the all-important blueprint set of chromosomes. Even if it succeeds to that point, older eggs have higher rates of replication errors that then introduce genetic problems. Each of these situations usually results in miscarriage. Perhaps because of these increased abnormalities, the success of the next step – implantation – is reduced to half by age 40. If an embryo *is* implanted, older women show a decreased ability to maintain a pregnancy.

Predicting the onset of menopause

While the average age at menopause is 51, this can range from 40 to 60 years of age. Thus, women who go through menopause earlier than average would have a miscarriage rate similar to older women. For example, if a woman will go through menopause 10 years early, her chance of successful pregnancy at 39 might be roughly equivalent to the miscarriage rate of a 49-year old. Conversely, women who will go through menopause later than average enjoy success rates typical of younger women.

Much research is being done to develop reliable predictors for menopause, and alternatives should become increasingly available.

For example, Australian researchers have shown that menstrual diaries can help predict menopause up to two years before it occurs (although this method cannot be used if you are on the birth control pill or any other medication that artificially regulates or suppresses your cycle.) The researchers found that variability of cycle length is the norm, but that a marked increase in this variability can indicate that the menopausal transition has begun. Variability, or "running range," is calculated as the difference between the shortest and longest cycle lengths. For example, if the shortest cycle (measured from the onset of one menstrual period to the onset of the next) is 21 days, and the longest is 35 days, then the running range is 14 days. During a woman's reproductive years her running range of cycle lengths is changing only slowly. However, when the running range first exceeds 42 days, it is beginning to increase quite quickly. This indicates that the menopausal transition has begun, and a woman is unlikely to have more than 20 more menstrual cycles.

Elsewhere, researchers in Britain have found they can predict the onset of menopause by evaluating a woman's age, her hormone levels, and the size of her ovaries as measured by ultrasound.

Infertility

Most of us think of infertility and miscarriage as separate issues, and they often are; infertility can be due to a number of causes that have nothing to do with miscarriage. However, there are circumstances when "miscarriage" and "infertility" can be two ways of describing the same thing.

Miscarriages that occur prior to confirmation of a pregnancy (in steps 1-3 at the beginning of this chapter: fertilization, replication, and implantation) are essentially "invisible miscarriages" in the sense that a woman doesn't yet know she's pregnant. When she gets her period on time, it is evidence of infertility – but it is also an unseen miscarriage. This distinction is important because women – especially older women – are bombarded with bad news about infertility and miscarriage. The obstacles can seem overwhelming when we read that infertility increases with age, that older eggs are associated with increased problems in fertilization, replication, and implantation, and that older women have higher miscarriage rates in very early pregnancy. But these are just three ways of saying the very same thing. While the challenges that older women face are real, they must be kept in their proper perspective – what appears to be multiple problems can often be just one.

Are miscarriage rates increasing?

In order to answer this question we need to compare only two things: the current miscarriage rate and the miscarriage rate at some time in the past.

But even the first part of the equation presents a challenge. As discussed at the beginning of this chapter, two different experts could quote current miscarriage rates of 75% and 20% – and both would be right! The only difference is that the first would be talking about the chance of miscarriage for a fertilized egg, and the second would be quoting the miscarriage rate of confirmed pregnancies.

Today there is more dialogue than ever before about miscarriage and still it can seem impossible to tease out the facts. This challenge becomes insurmountable when looking at miscarriage data of 20 or 30 years ago – it does not exist in any form that can be reliably utilized. So although determining what is happening with miscarriage rates requires little information, it is not yet available. Thus, while this is currently a hotly debated topic, there is surprisingly little data behind any of the arguments. We cannot yet say if the real rate of miscarriage is increasing, decreasing, or remaining stable.

What *is* increasing, however, is the *incidence* of miscarriage. This is different than the *rate* of miscarriage. "Incidence" refers to how often something is detected; "rate" is how likely it is to occur at any given time. As an example of this difference, let's look at two factors that have increased the *incidence* of miscarriage even while the *rate* of miscarriage may have remained unchanged:

Increasing maternal age at first birth. In 1970 the average age of first-time mothers was 24.6 years old. By 2000 that had increased nearly three years, to 27.2 years of age. As we have seen, maternal age plays a significant role in miscarriage rate. So even if the miscarriage *rate* is unchanged (i.e. even if the chance of miscarriage at any given age is exactly the same in 2000 as it was in 1970), we would expect to see a higher *incidence* (i.e. a higher number) of miscarriages with this increase in average age, simply because 27-year olds miscarry more frequently than 24-year olds.

Improved availability and sensitivity of pregnancy tests. As miscarriage rates are so high early in pregnancy (especially before the first period is due), we would expect to see far more *incidence* of pregnancy loss as tests are developed that confirm pregnancies earlier and earlier. To use an extreme example, if there were a reliable test that confirmed the presence of a fertilized egg, then we could see the *incidence* of pregnancy loss rocket to 75%, even if the chance of a miscarriage occurring at any given stage of gestation hadn't changed at all – we would simply be getting a snapshot of a different part of the Miscarriage Rate chart shown previously.

So while the *incidence* of miscarriage is increasing, it is not cause for alarm; there are good reasons we would expect to see exactly this result even if the chance of miscarriage has not changed at all. Until we can compare reliable miscarriage data over a period of time, we cannot know if the actual chance of having a miscarriage is increasing, decreasing, or remaining stable.

Should women expect to miscarry at least once?

Many experts have said "most women should expect to miscarry at some stage." We can only hope this statement is intended to provoke thought rather than fear – to illustrate how common miscarriage really is. But is it true? That depends on how many children you plan on having. Because if you plan on getting pregnant only once, your chance of success is about 80% – although miscarriage is a common outcome, you certainly don't need to "expect" it. If you plan on four pregnancies, however, you would be in the minority if you did not experience at least one miscarriage.

Currently, the average number of children born to a woman in the US is 2.1 (or 210 children for every 100 women). The table below illustrates how the chance of having a miscarriage is influenced by the number of pregnancies a woman has. Based on the simplifying notion that one in every five pregnancies ends in miscarriage, statistics predict that:

- For every 100 women who get pregnant twice: the majority (64 of them) will never miscarry, nearly one-third (32 of them) will have one miscarriage, and four will have two.
- For every 100 women who get pregnant three times: a very slight majority (51 of them) will never miscarry, 38 will miscarry once, 10 of them twice, and one of them will miscarry three times.

Increasing Chance of Miscarriage with Multiple Pregnancies

NUMBER OF MISCARRIAGES	NUMBER OF PREGNANCIES: 1	2	3	4
0	80%	64%	51%	41%
1	20%	32%	38%	40%
2	-	4%	10%	15%
3	-	-	<1%	3%
4	-	-	-	<1%
Total	100%	100%	100%	100%

Therefore, while the average woman planning on having the average number of children needn't *expect* to miscarry, miscarriage remains a very common pregnancy outcome.

Sporadic versus recurrent miscarriage

Most miscarriages are "sporadic," meaning they are due to random chance. Even if a woman has several sporadic miscarriages, they are separate isolated events whose only link to each other is that they – coincidentally – happened to the same person.

Unlike sporadic miscarriage, "recurrent" miscarriage is caused by an underlying condition that increases the risk of the embryo being damaged, or of the womb being unable to provide adequate nourishment.

The difference between sporadic and recurrent miscarriage can be visualized by imagining a game spinner with an arrow and five segments. For most women, only one of the five segments will read "Miscarriage;" they have a one in five chance that – just by random chance – they will miscarry. By contrast, women with an underlying condition may have several segments that read "Miscarriage." It is highly unlikely that a woman have a 100% chance of miscarriage. This means that even without treatment, most women with an underlying problem will still be able to have children; they will just have a higher rate of miscarriage.

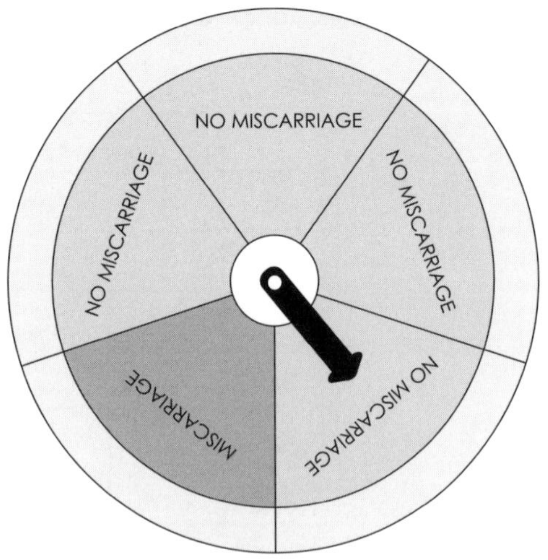

As an example, consider the case of a woman with a septate uterus (where the uterus is divided into two halves by a central wall, discussed in the chapter *Anatomical Abnormalities*). If the embryo implants on this middle wall with its relatively low blood supply, its needs will eventually outstrip the available nourishment, and miscarry. If, however, the embryo implants on the outer wall of the uterus, then the chance of miscarriage is no higher than for anyone else (though there may be problems later in the pregnancy). Assuming the embryo has an equal chance of implanting on the inner wall versus the outer wall, we would expect to see a miscarriage rate for this woman that was about twice as high as average.

"Sporadic" and "Recurrent" can be misleading

The difference between "sporadic" and "recurrent" can become confusing because of the way miscarriages are labeled. One miscarriage is automatically considered a sporadic miscarriage. (My doctor's terminology for a single sporadic miscarriage was "bad luck.") Two consecutive miscarriages (which my doctor called "very bad luck") are also automatically assumed to be sporadic. Three consecutive miscarriages are categorized as "recurrent miscarriage," and the woman termed a "recurrent miscarrier" (or more alarmingly, a "recurrent aborter").

Just reviewing the statistics of *sporadic* miscarriage: if each woman has a 20% (or one in five) chance of miscarrying a confirmed pregnancy, then about 25 women out of every 125 will have a sporadic miscarriage. Those 25 women will still have a 20% chance of sporadic miscarriage with their next pregnancy, and based on chance we would expect about five of them to have a second *sporadic* miscarriage. Of those five women, we would expect one of them (20%) to have a third consecutive *sporadic* miscarriage. This will be labeled "recurrent" miscarriage, though it is nothing more than very bad luck indeed.

Conversely, if a woman *does* have an underlying (or "recurrent") condition that puts her at greater risk of miscarriage, it is only her third miscarriage that will finally be classified as such. Her first and second miscarriages will automatically be labeled "sporadic."

Thus, as with any labeling based on statistics rather than on each individual to whom it is applied, the tags "sporadic" and "recurrent" can be misleading. The woman with a recurrent condition – whose first miscarriages will be labeled "sporadic" – may delay investigating the cause of her miscarriage until after her second or even third miscarriage. And the one in every 125 women who has three consecutive *sporadic* miscarriages will be termed a "recurrent miscarrier," and will likely be desperate for answers even though her miscarriages were caused by nothing more than being on the wrong end of the statistics.

Distinguishing sporadic from recurrent miscarriage

If a woman knew she had a condition that put her at higher risk of recurrent miscarriage, she would be unlikely to wait until she had lost three pregnancies before investigating. Likewise, if a woman who had three consecutive miscarriages could be *certain* it was due to nothing more than chance, then she would probably be able to approach her fourth pregnancy with a greater degree of calm. Unfortunately, without testing and investigation, there is no reliable way of telling whether a miscarriage was sporadic or due to recurrent causes. However, clues *can* often be gleaned upon closer inspection of the facts of the loss (for example, at what stage the pregnancy miscarried, whether there were any indications prior to the loss, whether there is a history of infertility, the particulars of other pregnancies, etc). This will be explored further in the chapter *Learning From Your Miscarriage History.*

Miscarriage causes

Miscarriage is caused when something interferes with any of the first four steps of pregnancy summarized earlier in this chapter (fertilization, replication, implantation, and growth). The chart below shows the relative proportion of conditions causing miscarriage. These conditions arise from chromosomal problems, immunological disorders, anatomical abnormalities, hormonal imbalance, and occasionally from other sources such as maternal infection. Each of these conditions – and how to test for and treat them – will be discussed in detail.

Miscarriage Causes

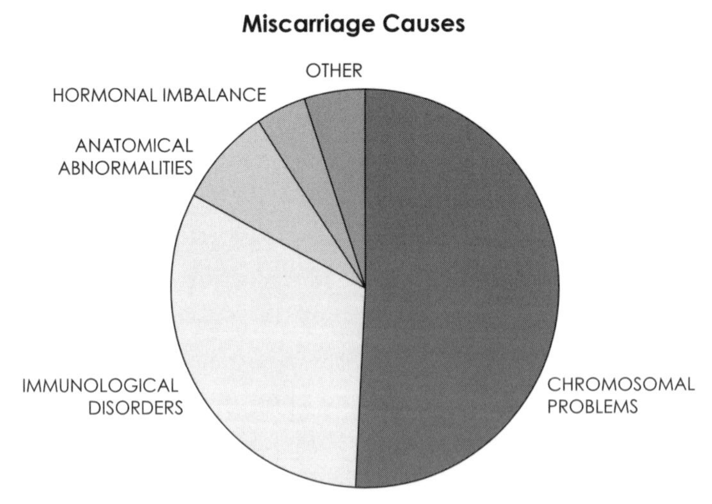

Why doctors are reluctant to investigate

While women have very good reasons for wanting to know exactly why they miscarried, doctors have good reasons for not wanting to investigate each miscarriage. Once again, this situation is simply the clash that occurs when statistics and averages are applied at a very personal, individual level. Each woman who miscarries wants to know the specific reasons for her loss, and to understand her particular outlook. But each doctor knows that *chances are* it was just bad luck. Specifically, doctors think twice about investigating miscarriage because doing so requires a great deal of time and energy and does not always produce an answer, and because miscarriage is a problem that usually solves itself:

The numbers are daunting. The average urban obstetrician-gynecologist could expect more than 50 of his patients to miscarry every year. While those women may all want to know the precise reason they miscarried, he cannot provide it unless he has found a specific answer, and finding such an answer is only possible through investigation. In a busy practice, doctors tend to resist testing, as they know that the great majority of cases will be due to nothing more than random chance.

Answers are hard to find. Historically, investigation provided an explanation in only about half of all cases. With increased knowledge and improved testing this "unexplained" portion continues to shrink, but many doctors are unaware of these diagnostic advances, or unconvinced of their benefits. Also, while investigation does not guarantee an answer, it does promise to be time consuming for both doctor and patient, and potentially costly, particularly if there are insurance difficulties.

Miscarriage usually solves itself. Most women will eventually carry a pregnancy to term so long as they are willing to keep trying. Even after three consecutive miscarriages, most women (55%) will go on to a successful pregnancy without any treatment.

What this means to you

As in the example of the septate uterus, most underlying conditions that put a woman at higher risk of miscarriage do *not* impact every pregnancy – they are "hit-or-miss." In that particular case, once implantation occurs on the outer uterine wall, the increased risk of miscarriage is removed. The good news is that even women with an underlying condition almost always have some chance of a healthy pregnancy, even without treatment. The bad news is that it also means recurrent miscarriage might not be promptly investigated, as the possibility of an underlying problem can often be dismissed based on a previous successful pregnancy.

It is therefore important *not* to rely only on population statistics and "accepted practice," but instead to use every available tool to determine your own miscarriage risk profile, and evaluate your own specific circumstances. The next chapters have been designed to help you do exactly that.

miscarriage myths and misinformation

Laura's story

We had our first child when I was 34. I didn't have any issues getting pregnant or in early pregnancy, but developed pre-eclampsia which got severe enough that I had to be hospitalized for several weeks at the end of my pregnancy. Andrew was delivered by caesarian-section at 38 weeks, which was as long as they wanted to let it go.

Two years later I was about nine weeks into my second pregnancy when we took Andy to Disneyland. It was an exhausting day of trekking all over the park in the heat. I ate what people eat at theme parks – hot dogs, hamburgers, popcorn, ice cream...

Just a day or two later I started bleeding heavily. I suspected right away that the day at Disneyland had caused me to miscarry. All that exertion, all that time on my feet, and all that junk food were the wrong things to do – especially in the first three months when my body needed rest. I felt like my body had to choose between me and the pregnancy, and it dumped the pregnancy – there was just too much physical stress to maintain it.

I didn't call the doctor or go to the hospital. There was never any question that it was a miscarriage. I hadn't seen a doctor yet about the pregnancy, and didn't think anything could be done. I thought there was nothing I could do except appreciate the healthy child I already had, and try again.

Even so, I had this huge sense of loss – like I'd had something precious and now I didn't. It didn't matter that I already had a child; I felt like I had lost someone. My reaction surprised me, and I think the fact that your hormones are all over the place only makes everything worse. I don't know how much of my reaction was driven by hormones.

After that first miscarriage I had another early miscarriage, but then I had our daughter Laura. Then I had a last early miscarriage before having Alexandra, who completed our family. So in the end I had three children and three miscarriages.

I know some people think miscarriage is nature's way of weeding out pregnancies with faulty genes, but I didn't see it as a blessing or a biological solution in any way. I felt like it didn't have to happen – like I lost a child I could have had. I think I could have prevented that loss if I had acted differently.

miscarriage myths and misinformation

It is human nature to want to get to the bottom of why bad things happen – especially something as devastating as miscarriage. While this is a worthy goal (and the main goal of this book), there are many things that are incorrectly blamed for causing early pregnancy loss.

It is natural to look back on the hours or days leading up to the miscarriage, searching for the cause. It is also natural to remember something that happened beforehand, and suspect it had something to do with the miscarriage. But much as it may seem logical to blame the incident (or yourself) for the miscarriage, this is almost never the cause. Experiencing bleeding after sex, or lifting something heavy and feeling a pain in your back, or having too many cocktails before you knew you were pregnant – even though they may have occurred just prior to the loss – do not cause healthy pregnancies to miscarry.

The fact is that miscarriages happen, no matter how much we may or may not want a baby, and no matter how much we may or may not do our best to prevent that miscarriage. Miscarriage is impartial in choosing victims, which is what makes it so frightening – it means it's hard to anticipate or control.

Despite the random nature of miscarriage, most women who experience one will question whether they did something to cause it. Some women even want to believe they did, in the hope they might be able to control the outcome the next time (e.g. "If I don't go to the gym next time, I won't miscarry," or "If I don't tell people I'm pregnant next time, I won't jinx it"). This self-incrimination may be a normal part of the process, but it's a destructive one, and is the reason this chapter is important. Berating yourself over something you didn't cause – and couldn't prevent – directs your energy against yourself, hindering your ability to move on and take positive action.

Because miscarriage is a subject still mostly reserved for private conversations, myths thrive in a relative absence of scrutiny. These misconceptions fuel post-miscarriage feelings of guilt, confusion, and powerlessness, all of which diminish our energy and effectiveness. The following are some of the most popular myths that contribute to women feeling they are to blame for their pregnancy loss. Not one of these myths is true.

Myth: It's all my fault – even the name says so!

I'll never forget telling my father I'd miscarried. "How'd you do that?" he wondered. (There is much to be said for having your partner, a sibling, or a friend break the news to people unable to support you in this difficult time.) While the directness of his response may have been unusual, the sentiment was not. The myth still flourishes that miscarriages are caused by something the woman did "wrong." Even the term "miscarried" suggests the baby was "mis-carried," as though the mother carelessly fumbled it. But nothing could be further from the truth.

The fact is that the most common cause of miscarriage is random chromosomal error. Once these errors occur (usually at the moment of conception), there is nothing a woman can do to save the pregnancy; and it is certainly not her fault when it miscarries. Of miscarriages that are due to other factors, most are completely out of anyone's control (e.g. a poorly formed umbilical cord).

It is worth bearing in mind that pregnancies are designed to weather the rough-and-tumble that life throws at them. The human race would have come to an end long ago if pregnancies couldn't withstand physical exertion, shock, stress, disease, or inadequate diet. Whatever activity you blame for your miscarriage probably pales in comparison with what our ancestors in the caves were putting their pregnancies through (where a happy day at Disneyland would have probably been the least physically demanding day of their lives!)

Myth: I miscarried from too much stress

The fact that some level of stress is inherent in all our lives – and is therefore common to virtually all women who miscarry – gives this myth its appeal. (Of course, stress is also common to all women who have successful pregnancies, but that gets overlooked.)

Every woman worries about something during pregnancy. Many women feel under pressure at some time in pregnancy. Some experience trauma, shock, or extreme anxiety during pregnancy (such as the death of a family member, loss of a job, or news that a loved one has a terminal illness). And yet, somehow these women survive all this negative energy. And so do their babies.

As an extreme example, more than 100 babies were born whose fathers were killed in the terrorist attacks of September 11, 2001. These babies were at all different stages of gestation when their fathers were killed (many men didn't even know their wives were pregnant). And yet those women – and those babies – went on to survive some of the most harrowing, stressful circumstances possible.

The greatest threat posed by stress is if it results in a woman adopting dangerous coping behavior (e.g. she is unable to eat properly for most of the pregnancy, or engages in heavy smoking, drinking, or drug taking).

Also, women with high blood pressure ("hypertension") or other conditions that may restrict blood flow to the developing embryo will need to actively manage these disorders, as stress can aggravate these conditions (e.g. by raising blood pressure further), and harm both mother and baby if not controlled.

Myth: It's because I wasn't sure I wanted a baby

This is a myth fraught with guilt, and is therefore one of the most harmful. There is not a shred of truth to this myth.

It is perfectly normal to worry about how the baby will impact your life, your relationship, your work, your friendships, and your body. It is also normal to have misgivings (whether minor or major) about having a baby. Your attitude to the pregnancy does not impact whether it lives or dies. If willpower determined the fate of pregnancy, then women who long desperately for a child would never suffer the devastation of miscarriage, and rape victims would never require a termination. Much as we would like for our wishes to dictate the course life takes, we know life doesn't always work that way – often things happen without any regard to our own thoughts or wishes. Miscarriage is one of those things.

Myth: It's a sign I'm not fit to be a mother

Miscarriage is a phenomenon that doesn't discriminate between "good" and "bad" mothers. But while miscarriage is definitely *not* caused by a woman's destiny to be an unfit mother, it may actually have the reverse effect on her future parenting. Women who have suffered a miscarriage report that their children (whether future or existing) become even more precious to them. These women find they parent more patiently and constructively, and are less likely to take their children for granted.

Myth: There must be something wrong with me

On the contrary, a miscarriage is considered by doctors to be a good sign! It means that your body has mastered the difficult parts of the process, which are fertilization and implantation. In fact, if the pregnancy was chromosomally flawed, as is the case with most miscarriages, then your body was working exactly as it is designed to.

Chromosomal errors found in the great majority of miscarriages tend to be random, and are unlikely to recur. For miscarriages that were not due to chromosomal abnormality, there are many reasons that have nothing to do with you that could result in a loss. For example, at implantation the fertilized egg bores into the uterine lining. In doing so, it sends tiny offshoots to connect to the maternal blood supply. If these offshoots or their connections are faulty, the pregnancy will be unable to survive.

Myth: The baby must have had a problem

While this is often the case, it is not necessarily so. There are many factors that can cause healthy embryos to miscarry. Some of these factors are created by the pregnancy itself, and are unlikely to be repeated (as mentioned in the previous myth). Some factors, however, may result from an underlying problem with the mother, which makes them likely to happen again – it is these miscarriage risk factors that are addressed in this book.

Myth: I miscarried because I overdid it

Before becoming pregnant, many women imagine pregnancy as a sort of "Madonna-and-child" scenario (all peaceful golden glow, set to a soaring symphony). The reality is usually very different. Nausea, fatigue, and the endless list of things to do before the baby arrives can make would-be Madonnas feel as though they are Madonna the singer: overscheduled, overcommitted, and overtaxed. As Laura found, even a day at Disneyland can feel like a major struggle. Nonetheless, much as life's frenetic pace and constant demands may make us feel wrung out, the embryo floats through it all in relative peace and harmony, just enjoying the ride.

Myth: I miscarried because I didn't eat properly

Particularly in early pregnancy, the developing baby will take whatever nutrients it needs from your body. If you have an inadequate intake of calcium, for example, the baby will leach it from your bones. In early pregnancy, your eating habits are largely to protect your own health!

Of course, if your diet is unhealthy throughout pregnancy, there can be harm to the developing baby, whose nutritional requirements increase with growth and development. But when considering miscarriage in the first 20 weeks of pregnancy, eating habits simply do not cause pregnancy loss.

Myth: I'm too fat (or too thin) to carry a baby

Unless you are dangerously fat (obese), dangerously thin, or in some cases a dedicated athlete, weight just isn't part of the equation.

If you are obese

Obese women do have significantly higher risk of first trimester miscarriage than women in the normal weight range. In addition, "severely obese" women have a significantly higher miscarriage rate than "obese" women. Thus, doctors point out that losing even some weight can markedly improve a woman's odds of successful pregnancy.

If you are a dedicated athlete

Body fat plays a key role in conception and pregnancy, and if your body fat is too low (elite athletes or dedicated runners can fall into this category), it can result in irregular menstrual cycles, or no menstrual period at all.

If you have regular cycles and you are ovulating, this is a good indication that your weight and body fat are not too low to conceive and carry a pregnancy to term. Where female athletes do not have regular cycles, reducing training and increasing weight have been shown to dramatically improve successful pregnancy outcomes.

If you are underweight

As with athletes, maintaining adequate body fat will be of concern for women who are underweight. If you have simply always been slender (or "slight," or "small-boned," or whatever term you prefer) and your monthly cycle is regular, then that's likely the way you were designed, and of no concern.

If, however, you are abnormally underweight, then it is the condition causing this that could increase your miscarriage risk. For example, women with eating disorders are at risk of depriving their pregnancies of the nourishment required for normal development. Women suffering from serious diseases have a higher risk of miscarriage arising from the disease itself (e.g. by interfering with hormone production) or from side-effects of treatment or medication.

If you are underweight and have had difficulty conceiving or carrying a pregnancy, then addressing and correcting any underlying conditions that may exist, and putting on some weight, can give you much better odds of a successful pregnancy.

Myth: I miscarried because I continued to exercise

Staying active actually *helps* you and the baby. While it is essential to work with your doctor or health care professional to tailor an exercise regime to meet your specific circumstances, routine exercise helps keep you strong and flexible, and maintains your stamina (all of which will come in handy in labor, or when chasing a toddler). In addition, regular exercise appears to lower the risk of developing gestational diabetes by increasing insulin sensitivity.

If you are an athlete, or following a more rigorous training regimen, it is worth speaking to your doctor about your specific program. Aspects you need to monitor include body fat (discussed in the previous myth), impact, body temperature and heart rate.

Impact. This refers to how much jolt your body has to absorb: swimming and walking are low-impact; running is high-impact; and pole vaulting, horse jumping, and skydiving are eye-poppingly high-impact. In very early pregnancy the embryo can weather almost anything you can, but as the pregnancy progresses, impact poses an increasing risk.

Body temperature. Body temperature increases with exercise – the more intense the exercise, the higher your core temperature (this rises even more if you are unfit, dehydrated, exercising for prolonged periods, or exercising in a hot environment). Increased core body temperature is not associated with miscarriage, but birth defects have been linked to temperatures above 102°F (39°C) that are sustained for more than 24 hours. Most exercise does not pose any problem.

Heart rate. As your heart rate increases with exercise, there is a decrease in blood flow to the developing baby. However, this is offset (and oxygen levels maintained) because fetal heart rate also increases. Though you should discuss your specific circumstances with your doctor, it is generally thought that keeping heart rate at or under 140 beats per minute is optimal (this should be kept even lower if you are unfit or over 40).

Myth: I miscarried because I lifted something heavy

Pregnancy is no different from any other time in the sense that lifting – whether it's weights at the gym or children at home – should be done properly (i.e. with adequate positioning and support). But harming the pregnancy by lifting is unlikely, as your body reacts to the pain and makes you drop whatever you're lifting before you can strain yourself enough to do damage to the pregnancy.

If lifting weights at the gym, isolate the arms or legs doing the lifting (you shouldn't feel it through the rest of your body). If lifting at home, squat and lift using the large muscles in your legs, rather than lifting by bending over and straining the weaker muscles in your back. Doing this improperly is still not a risk for miscarriage, but because of the extra demands placed on your body during pregnancy, sore backs take longer to recover.

Myth: I miscarried from a blow to my stomach

A woman's body is designed to shield the developing baby from physical harm. The earlier the pregnancy – and the smaller the embryo – the more unlikely it is to be impacted by external bumps and thumps. For example, at two months the embryo is smaller than a walnut. It floats peacefully in the amniotic fluid in the amniotic sac, protected from pokes and jolts. The amniotic sac, in turn, is cushioned by the womb. To injure or dislodge the pregnancy would require a blow severe enough to damage internal organs.

However, as the pregnancy progresses, several things happen that reduce the fetus's protection: the baby itself grows and begins to protrude from the woman's body; the uterine wall thins as it stretches, and the amniotic sac – which was a roomy, protective environment in early pregnancy – stretches until it provides only a small cushion by the end of term. In addition, late in pregnancy the baby and placenta begin to have significant weight and size of their own, and may move differently than the rest of a woman's body in the event of a physical shock (e.g. in a car accident a woman's seatbelt might hold her securely in place, but the placenta could be wrenched by the impact).

Injuries, knocks, or jolts to your abdominal area are usually of no concern in early pregnancy, and are highly unlikely to cause miscarriage. But these same knocks become more serious as your pregnancy progresses. If they are the kind that result from having toddlers at home (all sharp knees and flailing elbows, desperate for a cuddle), then they are probably of little consequence. But if they are the result of anything more sinister (intentional abuse from anyone), then they should be considered life threatening to your baby, as abuse that wouldn't harm an embryo at two months could kill a fetus at seven months. (Distressingly, many women report that their partner's violence began when they were first pregnant, or markedly increased when they were pregnant.) If you are in a situation of abuse, try to draw courage to take action from knowing that you are the protector not only of yourself, but of your baby.

Myth: Sex caused my miscarriage

Perhaps it's only logical to think that because sex has the power to begin a pregnancy, it also has the power to end one. It doesn't. (At least, not in early pregnancy. Because orgasm causes the uterus to contract, there is a theory that this could coax the body into labor when the baby approaches full term. I know many couples that tested this premise for weeks as their due dates came and went; they all agree that while it made the waiting more enjoyable, it had no impact whatever. While some women may experience painful contractions after orgasm, this does not lead to premature delivery.)

Of course, because sex is one of the few activities that comes anywhere close to the developing baby, it is often suspected as the cause of a miscarriage. However, sex (even the passionate kind, and even with the most well-endowed man) only penetrates the vagina, while the baby is safely tucked away way up in the uterus, past the closed cervix. Because the cervix is soft and filled with blood, however, some thumping during sex can sometimes cause it to bleed a little (which will result in spotting), but this is not a problem.

To harm the baby, something would have to get *past* the cervix. This would require the cervix to dilate, which is painful (and would instantly douse any desire to continue). But even that would not be enough; harming the baby would require scraping or suctioning the uterine wall, or introducing a serious disease into the uterine cavity.

While fears that sex will cause miscarriage, fetal damage, or even premature labor are very common, studies have shown there is no significant increase in any of these things in women who continue to be sexually active throughout pregnancy.

Myth: I miscarried because I once had an abortion

Several studies have shown that elective abortion does not increase a woman's risk of miscarriage in the future.

Elective termination of pregnancy (i.e. an abortion) is performed via D&C (dilation and curettage, discussed at length in the chapter *Miscarriage Management*). This is exactly the same procedure used to empty the uterus of the "products of conception" after miscarriage, and there should be no damage or scarring to the uterus or cervix. Within a few weeks your body should be able to sustain a pregnancy as though the abortion never occurred. This is the case regardless of whether you've had one or many abortions.

Myth: I miscarried because I just went off the pill

The myth that women should discontinue using birth control pills several months before conception has no basis in fact. On the contrary, studies have indicated that, if anything, the risk of miscarriage is slightly lower for women who have used the pill.

There are a number of justifications cited for going off the pill several months before conception, including the increased risk of twins, irregular periods as your body gets "back to normal," and potential harm to the baby from birth control hormones.

Discontinuing the birth control pill just prior to conception does increase the odds of ovulating more than one egg. However, only about one in every 40 women who gets pregnant right after discontinuing the pill will have twins, compared to about one in 80 women who were not on the pill. Depending upon your desire to avoid or have twins, this might represent a risk or an opportunity.

Irregularity is cited as a problem because of the concern that it could make it more difficult to accurately date the pregnancy, or to become pregnant in the first place. Of course, due dates are more accurately predicted using ultrasound, whether a woman is regular or not. In addition, the pill has not been shown to cause any delay in becoming pregnant. On the contrary, some women with hormonal imbalance find that the pill corrects the problem for a few months, and *need* to use it until just prior to becoming pregnant. If these women were to wait for three months before becoming pregnant, the corrective influence would be completely lost.

As for harming the baby with high levels of toxic hormones, that is simply not the case. Aside from the fact that the hormones in birth control pills (progesterone and/or estrogen) occur naturally in your body, the small amounts in birth control pills are completely cleared from your body in a matter of days. This is why you are advised to use alternative birth control if you ever forget to take the pill for two days in a row. In addition, birth control pills work by preventing ovulation; they do not prevent implantation, growth, or development. Even if you accidentally continued taking the pill after you were already pregnant, it would not be expected to affect the pregnancy.

Myth: It's my own fault for waiting so late

My most painful loss was – thankfully – also my last. It was my only pregnancy with a genetic disorder – a rare syndrome "incompatible with life." Just afterwards, a grandmother (incorrectly) charged, "Well what did you expect? The chance of having a Down's Syndrome child is one in 10 at your age." At my age (which was 38) the chance of having a Down's Syndrome child was actually one in 190. By my calculations, the chance of having the disorder our embryo actually had was one in 80,000. But even if my chance of success *had* been slim, the implication that failure was deserved was unwarranted and unhelpful.

While delaying childbearing does increase the risk of miscarriage, it does not mean you *deserve* one. This myth implies you were so irresponsible (or "selfish") that your miscarriage is simply life's way of putting you back in your place.

It is worth remembering that women who delay childbearing usually do so in order to achieve a better balance in their lives (e.g. finish their education, find the right life partner, build a resilient career, achieve financial wellbeing, etc). This benefits not only themselves, but their children; we may be at the lowest risk of miscarriage in our early 20s, but few of us would be the best mothers we could be at that age. Studies have shown that older mothers are likely to be more calm, relaxed, patient, and confident. They are also more likely to make time to enjoy their child, and are better at encouraging speech and independence in the child (in fact, reading scores for children of older mothers are higher than for children of younger mothers).

Whatever your reasons for waiting, they were the right reasons for you, and it is admirable to manage your life to try to achieve the best balance. While these choices may increase your risk of miscarriage, they do not mean you deserve one, or that you don't deserve children. And perhaps these same choices will make your home a happier one when you do become a mother.

Myth: Nobody knows what I'm going through

While there are a great many women who lose pregnancies, not a single one will feel it exactly as you do. However, this does not mean you have to go through the experience alone. While no one else will be exactly like you, there will be others whose thoughts, feelings, or experiences with miscarriage resonate with you. There are many, many people who can potentially provide comfort and understanding: friends, family, colleagues, and professional counselors (grief counselors, psychologists, help lines, etc). Many other people are available to you on the Internet and through pregnancy loss support groups of various kinds. There are also many books dealing with the grief of miscarriage, which may help you overcome some of the issues arising from pregnancy loss.

While no one is exactly like you, there are many other people who have had the same experience; some of them may offer insights that help reduce your feelings of isolation. So although you may feel like withdrawing into yourself, if you can make yourself reach out to others who can help, and allow them to do so, you will benefit enormously. (See the chapter *The Power of Love.*)

Myth: My partner doesn't understand the pain I feel

Husbands can be funny that way. It's sometimes hard to know how they're feeling about losing the pregnancy. And because the pregnancy was never physically a part of them, women often assume their partners are less impacted by the loss.

While some men do find it hard to "bond" with a child before they see, hear, or feel tangible evidence (e.g. seeing the fetus in an ultrasound, hearing the heartbeat on a Doppler, or feeling the baby kick), others bond right from the start. And of course, it is only natural that men wonder in exactly the same way as women about how a baby will change their lives. So, like women, they can progress from fundamental questions of how they will cope, to imagining time they will share with this child, in a relatively short space of time. When the pregnancy is lost, they lose those dreams just as the woman does. However, they might show it in entirely different ways. This can be due to their own nature, and the way they grieve, or because they don't want their own sorrow to add to their wife's pain. While these men may go about their lives as though nothing happened, they often wait until they're alone (in the car, tool shed, or shower) to shed their tears.

Men and women often have more in common in their reaction to a pregnancy loss than they suspect. Even if they fundamentally disagreed about the pregnancy itself (e.g. one of them wanted a termination), they may both mourn the loss terribly, with the disapproving partner feeling guilty that negative feelings were somehow responsible for the loss.

Couples that can work through this experience together report that not only are they able to move on more quickly, but also that it strengthens their relationship. They understand each other better, and trust and rely on each other more. (For a more complete discussion of this subject, and how to work together with your husband to forge a stronger partnership in the face of miscarriage, see the chapter *Understand Your Partner*.)

Myth: I have to wait six months before trying again

Although it is "common knowledge" that couples should wait three, or six, or 12 months (depending on the source) before trying again to become pregnant, this is a myth for all but a very few women with specific physical complications such as a blood clot requiring medication or damage to the uterine wall. (If this is the case, then as with any physical condition your doctor diagnoses, you should be given full details of why the condition is suspected, how long it will take to heal, and how it will impact future pregnancies.) The great majority of women will find their body rebounds quickly after a miscarriage, and they can ovulate (and therefore become pregnant) as soon as two weeks later. There is no evidence to suggest that getting pregnant right away after a miscarriage increases the risk of having another.

This myth, however, is one that has its roots in good intentions: waiting can enable a date of conception to be more easily established for the next pregnancy, and it can allow a couple some time to recover emotionally.

Dating the next pregnancy

Because it's fine to resume sex as soon as the bleeding has stopped, it is possible to become pregnant again before the first post-miscarriage period; in this instance, the precise due date might not be clear. Of course, modern technology has made this virtually irrelevant, as an ultrasound scan is more accurate at predicting the baby's due date than the old method of counting cycle days anyway. Although it is still given as a reason to wait after a miscarriage, it should not influence your decision about what is best for you personally.

Emotional recovery

Although the physical effects wear off quickly, the psychological effects of a miscarriage can linger. Traditionally, doctors prescribed a waiting period in order to give their patients time to grieve.

While many women (though not all) will find they need a grieving period for the lost pregnancy, it is the couple – rather than the doctor – who should decide what is appropriate for them in their particular circumstances. For example, a 39-year old woman who had taken 13 months to get pregnant was prescribed a "routine" six-month wait by her doctor. She decided, however, that it would be better for her own recovery to continue trying – losing time only made her miscarriage feel more demoralizing and costly.

Of course, it is best if subsequent pregnancies are undertaken only when the couple feels resilient enough to cope with the possibility of success (and a baby), or failure (and another miscarriage). Recovery is very personal, and depends upon your unique character and circumstances. Don't let anyone try to tell you what is "normal" in this instance; it is whatever works best for you in balancing the need to grieve with the need to move on. Whether that means taking time out for a full grieving period, throwing yourself into the next pregnancy, or anything in between, you are the person best able to make that choice.

Myth: Now I'm more likely to miscarry again

One of the most frightening aspects of miscarriage is that it throws our reproductive future into doubt. Of course, the simple fact is that the reproductive process is highly complex and often fails; perfectly healthy women with no underlying condition will experience miscarriage at the rate of 20%, or one in five.

Most likely, you are among the great majority of women with no underlying condition, and are no more likely to miscarry your next pregnancy than anyone.

But if you *do* have a condition that will pose a risk to each pregnancy, then it existed before you ever had a miscarriage; the miscarriage was only a symptom of the problem, not the cause. The miscarriage itself does not increase your chance of having another – your chance is exactly the same as it was before. On the contrary, if a miscarriage can assist you in identifying an underlying condition and getting it treated, then that miscarriage actually helped *increase* your odds of the next pregnancy being a successful one.

While it may sound surprising, many experts believe that a miscarriage is an excellent sign that things are working. Getting pregnant is actually more difficult than staying pregnant; couples that miscarry have already demonstrated that they can do the harder part of the process, and usually go on to success in subsequent pregnancies. It is reported that 97% of couples who suffer a miscarriage end up being parents.

Instead of seeing a miscarriage as something that dooms future pregnancies, perhaps we should try to see it as an opportunity to improve our chance of future success.

Myth: I have a child, so can't have a problem

Not true. Some people win the lottery the first time they buy a ticket, some women find their life partner in their first boyfriend, and sometimes the right house is the first one you look at. Women with a problem that makes them likely to experience recurrent miscarriage may have a trouble-free pregnancy the first time they try. Women with an underlying disorder may have the reverse odds as normal women: four chances of miscarriage for every one chance of success. While these women will experience four times as many miscarriages as most women, they still have a chance of successful pregnancy, and may be lucky enough to achieve that the first time (and thereafter, if their luck continues to hold).

Myth: Next time I won't tell anyone I'm pregnant

Despite believing there is no such thing as "jinxes," many of us still prefer not to "tempt fate" by announcing a pregnancy too soon. Another reason this myth has some appeal is that about 95% of all miscarriages happen in the first three months. Waiting until after the high-risk period is over should save us from having to explain to people that we miscarried, if that turns out to be the result.

While this sounds logical, it turns out to be misguided, as I discovered. I decided not to tell anyone other than my husband when I became pregnant after a miscarriage, thinking it would spare me having to break bad news if it ended badly. Unfortunately, it did end badly, and I realized the flaw in this strategy. What I needed then was support and understanding from my nearest and dearest. While my husband was supportive, he had also suffered the loss and I didn't want him to be responsible for providing my sole support. I wanted my mother, my sister, and my best friends to support me, and knew they would give me the solace I needed. But those were odd phone calls, where I had to tell them I'd lost a pregnancy they hadn't even known about. They were disconnected from it, much as none of us wanted it to be that way. They hadn't hoped along with me each day, celebrated a little more each week, and then been shocked by the loss when it came. Because I hadn't lived the pregnancy with them, I hadn't been able to share my joys, and in the end I wasn't able to share the burden of my loss. Not telling my "support group" robbed us all of a chance to connect. "Sparing" friends and family sounded noble, but was unwise.

In fact, having a good support group is so essential that it is covered extensively in the chapter *The Power of Love;* support can make a great difference to how happy you are through pregnancy, and may even increase your chance of success.

Summary

Although we often fear a miscarriage was our own fault, this is practically never the case. Despite all the myths, there is almost nothing we can do to make a healthy pregnancy miscarry in the first 20 weeks. Unfortunately, there is almost nothing we can do to save a non-viable pregnancy or to prevent an inevitable miscarriage, either. And while each of us will experience guilt, struggle, and acceptance in different measures, ceasing to accuse ourselves is a vital step in moving forward toward a better future.

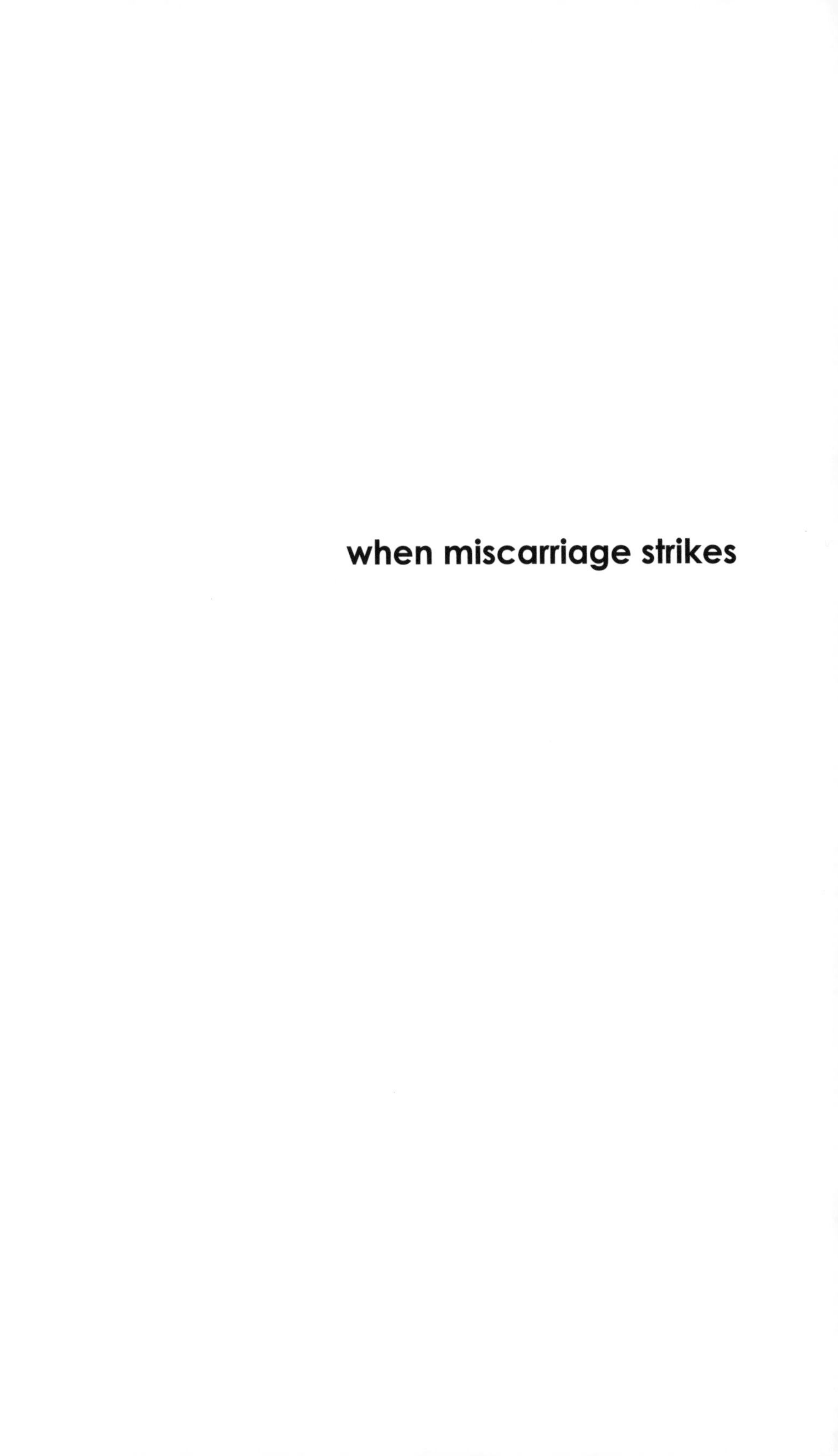

when miscarriage strikes

could it be miscarriage?

My story

I knew I was pregnant before I missed my period. I'd been pregnant – and miscarried – before, and knew just how it felt. For me, the "dishwasher test" is more accurate than a pregnancy test: if we forget to run the dishwasher at night, then when I open it the next morning I vomit instantly if I'm pregnant.

I was all scrubbed up and dressed for work when I opened the dishwasher to load my breakfast dishes. One whiff of that stale air and I threw up. My husband was just coming downstairs, and taking in the sight of me retching into the kitchen sink, asked with some alarm whether I was okay. "I'm okay," I said, "Just pregnant." And I was.

I was wary about the pregnancy holding, as we'd miscarried four times already. The first few weeks were especially nerve wracking, and I dreaded going to the bathroom, in case I'd find I was starting to miscarry. Then one day, I saw I was spotting. The shock of that image is still sharp.

But the spotting lasted only a day or two. The dishwasher test still worked (we often forgot to run it), and the pregnancy continued. Of course, after that I really dreaded going to the bathroom, scared it might happen again. And a couple of weeks later, it did. By then I was eight or nine weeks along, which was in the timeframe I had lost the previous pregnancies.

Since the pregnancy had already survived one episode of bleeding, I tried to be calm. On the other hand, the pregnancy was further along, and I was under the impression that bleeding is more worrisome the further along it is in pregnancy. Also, I was at a "high risk" stage according to my previous history, and could only wonder why this pregnancy kept bleeding – was it doomed to fail?

But that round of bleeding was just like the previous one – it lasted a day or two and then it stopped. So despite thinking things were looking grim, everything was absolutely fine. I had a perfectly normal (or if anything, abnormally easy) pregnancy after that, and delivered my first child – a beautiful baby boy – at full term.

could it be miscarriage?

Unfortunately, more than a million American women suffer a miscarriage every year. Perhaps a million more wonder whether they might lose their pregnancy. When I had symptoms that concerned me I wanted information about them, reassurance, and suggestions for appropriate action. This chapter aims to provide all three.

Why reading the signs becomes so important

For most of us there are very few moments in early pregnancy when we really know what is going on with the developing baby. At a doctor's appointment we may hear the baby's heartbeat; at certain stages of the pregnancy we might even get to see an ultrasound. But these events occur only a handful of times in an entire pregnancy. Until the baby starts moving on its own, there is little regular indication of whether the pregnancy is proceeding normally. Thus, it is no surprise that women search for any sign that might indicate how their pregnancy is progressing. And because that is all there is to go on, these signs can take on undeserved significance.

Signs that may worry you

Comparing your pregnancy with anyone else's – even your own previous pregnancies – can lead to needless worry. Because every woman and every baby is different, every pregnancy is different. For example, I had terrible morning sickness with my son, and no morning sickness with my daughter. Although they were completely different, both pregnancies were successful. Similarly, women with identical symptoms can have different outcomes.

Listed below are symptoms that can make women worry about the health of their pregnancy.

Bleeding or "spotting"

While vaginal bleeding in the first three months of pregnancy can often be a normal part of the process, it invariably causes alarm. Even more worrying, medical professionals refer to this bleeding as a "threatened miscarriage" or (worse still) a "threatened abortion." Concerns are that the placenta could be degrading or detaching from the side of the womb, or that the body could be shedding the failed pregnancy. Rarely, there could be an ectopic pregnancy (when the pregnancy implants outside the uterus), or a molar pregnancy (when the placenta acts like a cancer). Bleeding can occasionally indicate a hormone deficiency, or a vaginal or cervical infection. In general, the heavier the bleeding is, the more worrisome it is.

Symptoms: Any discharge of blood from the vagina, ranging from brown to bright red, and from spotting (occasional drops of blood) to heavy bleeding.

The good news: The fact is that while about one in four women (20% to 30%) will experience vaginal bleeding in the first 20 weeks of pregnancy, the vast majority of these women (70% to 80%) will continue their pregnancies and have healthy babies at full term. The odds are stacked in your favor on other major risk factors, as well: the risk of ectopic pregnancy is only about one in 200, and for molar pregnancy it is less than one in 1,500.

What to hope for: Bleeding may possibly result from the fertilized egg successfully implanting in the womb, or from the placenta embedding and developing in the uterine lining (both good things). Bleeding can be due to hormonal changes, and some women notice bleeding at the time they would normally have had their period. Because the cervix swells and softens in pregnancy, harmless bleeding can sometimes result from intercourse. And sometimes there is no identifiable reason for bleeding, with the pregnancy progressing normally to successful delivery.

When to consult a doctor: Although light spotting is not usually considered a major problem, it is worth speaking to your doctor, especially if bleeding persists or increases. Heavier bleeding, or bleeding paired with abdominal pain or other symptoms, requires immediate attention. If you cannot reach your doctor, contact a hospital emergency room.

Discharge of tissue or blood clots

The concern is that a miscarriage is in process, and that your body is expelling the embryo, placenta, or associated material (medically referred to as the "products of conception"). The prognosis for heavy blood flow accompanied by passage of clots or other material is not good. (If you do miscarry in early pregnancy, do not look for an actual embryo – it may look like a blood clot or lump with a small, disc-shaped placenta attached.)

Symptoms: Passage of clots or clumps from the vagina, accompanying vaginal bleeding. (Any discharged material should be collected in a sterile container if possible; see the next chapter for details.)

The good news: Passage of tissue during pregnancy does not always signal a miscarriage. Although the cause is unknown, a small amount of menstrual-like tissue can sometimes become loose and break away, passing out of the body and appearing to be a miscarriage. (This distressing phenomenon can also happen when a woman is not pregnant.)

What to hope for: If the tissue that is lost is simply a collection of tissue debris (such as part of the uterine lining independent of the embryo), then it can be of no consequence to your pregnancy.

When to consult a doctor: Discharge of clots or lumps requires immediate medical attention. If your doctor is unavailable, go to a hospital emergency room, and ensure that any material is collected in a sterile container, as it will need to be analyzed to determine whether it is simply debris, or actual pregnancy tissue.

Pelvic cramps, abdominal pain, or lower back pain

Your body stretches and reshapes itself throughout pregnancy in order to accommodate, protect and nourish your baby. Aches and pains – and even cramps – that come and go probably signify only that your body is changing (as it is supposed to) to meet the demands of your pregnancy. However, it causes concern because in early pregnancy cramps can be a sign of an ectopic pregnancy, or that the cervix is opening and that a miscarriage is imminent or underway. When abdominal pain is accompanied by bleeding the chance of it being a miscarriage increases.

Symptoms: Cramping or pain in the abdominal or pelvic areas, from light to severe, which may be accompanied by dizziness.

The good news: Though most women experience aches and pains at some time during pregnancy (and some women have them throughout), this is usually due to increased strain on the pregnant body, and does not signify a problem with the pregnancy.

When to consult a doctor: Even with mild pain, it is worth discussing your symptoms with your doctor. More intense pain, or pain that is accompanied by other symptoms, requires immediate attention.

Reduction or absence of symptoms of early pregnancy

Because pregnancy symptoms provide some of the only reassurance that early pregnancy is progressing, absence of these signs can lead to concerns about the health of the pregnancy.

Symptoms: Lack of signs of early pregnancy, including nausea (misnamed "morning sickness" though it often lasts all day), breast tenderness, general tiredness, and aches and pains.

The good news: Many women do not experience any of these symptoms. And while this may sound like a great piece of luck, the absence of physical discomfort also means an absence of proof that the pregnancy is progressing, and many women find this just as difficult to bear. Often it is only when they have progressed to the second or third trimester (or beyond) that women can look back happily upon their lack of discomfort in early pregnancy.

What to hope for: Various symptoms can come and go throughout a normal pregnancy. If you had a positive result on a reliable pregnancy test, but never had pregnancy symptoms, then there may be no cause for concern. If you had pregnancy symptoms that have diminished or disappeared, it could simply mean that they have passed (for example, many women stop having morning sickness toward the end of the first trimester, when pregnancy hormone levels taper off).

When to consult a doctor: If you did have symptoms of pregnancy and they have disappeared or diminished in a way you find worrying, then you should speak to your doctor about how to allay your fears – that is what he or she is there for.

A gush of fluid from the vagina

The amniotic sac protects and nourishes the fetus. A gush of fluid raises the concern that the sac has ruptured (a phenomenon most familiar as having your "waters break" when going into labor), which can make it impossible for the fetus to grow or develop, greatly increase the risk of infection, and cause miscarriage.

Symptoms: Sometimes fluid suddenly gushes from the vagina without bleeding or pain.

What to hope for: Small ruptures or tears in the amniotic sac early in pregnancy can often heal themselves, and the pregnancy can continue normally.

When to consult a doctor: Contact your doctor immediately, and watch for other symptoms (such as further leakage, bleeding, cramping, or fever). If none occur, and ultrasound indicates that the fetus is developing, then after a few days you may be able to return to normal activities.

What your doctor can do

Your doctor will likely have a great deal of previous experience with any symptoms that might be worrying you, and can probably provide you with the answers and support you need. Tests your doctor can use to determine the status of your pregnancy include ultrasound, confirmation of heartbeat, pelvic exam, blood test, analysis of any discharged material, and tests for infection:

Ultrasound (also called a "sonogram" or a "scan"). An ultrasound is the main test used when the status of a pregnancy is in doubt, as it can immediately determine the condition of the fetus, placenta, and uterus. More than 90% of first trimester pregnancies continue when a scan indicates that the baby is alive. There are no known harmful effects associated with the procedure (whether the probe is placed externally against the abdomen, or internally in the vagina), even when a woman is experiencing vaginal bleeding beforehand.

Confirmation of heartbeat. Heartbeat can be established on an ultrasound from six or seven weeks. It can also be detected using a hand-held monitor called a Doppler later in pregnancy. A Doppler bounces harmless sound waves off the fetal heart, which may be heard as early as nine or 10 weeks, depending upon the angle of the instrument, the position of the uterus, and how slim you are.

Pelvic examination. An internal exam can determine whether the cervix is opening (indicating a miscarriage), whether blood or other fluid is leaking from the cervix, whether the size of the uterus is appropriate for your stage of pregnancy, and whether any unusual lumps are present in the ovaries or fallopian tubes (to rule out the possibility of an ectopic pregnancy). More than one pelvic exam may be necessary over a period of hours or days to monitor changes.

Blood test. Measuring pregnancy hormone levels can sometimes be helpful in cases of suspected ectopic pregnancy or ambiguous ultrasound results. However, pregnancy hormone (called HCG for human chorionic gonadotropin) is produced by the placenta, and there is a huge range in normal levels. For example, the normal range for HCG at eight weeks is anywhere from 7,650 to 229,000 mIU/ml; at around 13 weeks it begins falling (which is why many women experience an easing of "morning sickness" toward the end of the first trimester). Without a previous test result, conclusions are hard to draw unless you actually lost the pregnancy some time ago (in which case the level of HCG should be below the normal range). Thus, in most cases this test will require two blood tests on different days to determine how hormone levels are changing.

Analysis of discharged material. Any material (clots or clumps) discharged from the vagina should be analyzed to determine whether it is "products of conception" (the fetus, placenta, etc). If so, then a miscarriage has occurred, and the doctor must then establish whether the miscarriage has been complete or partial. The material should be sent to a pathology lab with specific instructions to do chromosomal analysis, if possible (see the next chapter for further details.)

Tests for infection. Testing for vaginal or cervical infections may be appropriate, and a sample of vaginal secretions may be collected to determine whether amniotic fluid has been leaked, or whether infection is present.

If you feel you are about to miscarry

If you're afraid you might be about to miscarry, you can:

Call your doctor. Your doctor is an integral part of your pregnancy team, and it is his or her job (and wish) to help you. If you are concerned about the time of day or night, look to see if your doctor has an "after hours" number on his card or on his office answering machine. If so, there will be someone "on call." If you are truly worried about losing your pregnancy then the issue is one of life or death, and getting medical support at this time is naturally your first priority. Your doctor should arrange for you to have an ultrasound scan as soon as possible, which will almost always tell whether or not you have lost the pregnancy.

Speak to another trusted health professional. Whether it is your midwife, the technician who performed your ultrasound, or your cousin in medical school, they may be able to help you, especially if you are unable to reach your doctor. Do not worry about whether you are behaving "appropriately." People understand that women who fear they are losing a baby do not always call during office hours, make polite small talk, or have an appointment. They will likely do their utmost to help you.

Get assistance. If you do not get the attention or answers you need, then a visit to a hospital emergency room may be the best alternative.

Lie down. Many women notice that bleeding only occurs when they are standing up, so think that lying down stops it. In fact, your internal anatomy is something like a bottle – when you lie down the bottle is on its side, and fluids or tissue can only collect inside. Once you stand up the bottle is turned upside down and whatever has collected can flow out. It is therefore not surprising that lying down has not been shown to help; however, most of us feel better if we've done everything we could possibly do. So consider it a suggestion for your mind, more than anything else, as it may help you remain more focused and calm.

Can a miscarriage that has begun be averted?

By the time the body begins expelling a pregnancy, it has usually been dead for some time (often weeks). A miscarriage that has already begun (medically referred to as a "spontaneous abortion") is simply the body cleansing the uterus of material that is not going to result in a healthy baby, just as a menstrual period cleanses the uterus each month there is no pregnancy. Unfortunately, it is impossible to stop a miscarriage once the embryo or fetus has died, the cervix has dilated, or tissue has been lost.

Summary

Many women who experience bleeding, cramps, or other alarming signs worry that they might be losing their pregnancy. Happily, these fears are usually unfounded, and these women go on to deliver healthy babies.

If you do have a miscarriage, however, it can be a surprisingly difficult – even overwhelming – experience. But there are things you can do to answer some of the many questions that a miscarriage raises, and to mitigate some of the terrible feelings of guilt, loss, or lack of control you may feel. This will be discussed in the next chapter, *Miscarriage Management.*

miscarriage management

Collette's story

Everything had been going perfectly to plan: I met the man I wanted to share my life with, got engaged four months later, married five months after that, had the honeymoon, and got pregnant right away. I was coming up to my 37th birthday.

I had stopped working just before the wedding and planned to spend lots of time with my husband before the baby came along. But at 10½ weeks I had bleeding and pain that got worse through the weekend. On Sunday afternoon I called the doctor, who confirmed my fear that it could be a miscarriage. She told me that if it got worse I should call back, and that I might have to go to the hospital. Sunday night was very bad, with heavy bleeding and cramps; I feared the worst.

The next morning I had my first appointment with my obstetrician-gynecologist. He did an ultrasound, and confirmed that the baby was gone. He explained some things to me, though I felt numb and don't remember what. He scheduled me for a D&C that afternoon. That whole day is a hazy memory.

For the next week I went along on as though nothing significant had happened, but then reality set in and I finally cried. I cried the whole day.

I was pretty psychotic for about a month after the miscarriage. I got into nasty arguments about nothing with my husband and in-laws, who were visiting for Christmas. I couldn't believe I was reacting so strongly to the miscarriage. I kept thinking, "I'm strong, I can handle things, I got pregnant easily..." There were 51 reasons I thought I should be able to brush it off, but I couldn't. I hated having things taken out of my control. I wondered what I was doing with my life. I could handle not working while I was pregnant, because that put a time limit on how long I was sitting around doing nothing, but after the miscarriage it made me feel guilty and useless.

It took me a while to acknowledge that it's an upsetting thing, and that I shouldn't be angry at myself for being affected by it.

Luckily the uncertainty didn't last long; I found out I was pregnant about two months after the miscarriage.

I barely told a soul about that second pregnancy until I was four months along, and it was only once I was six months along that I really began to think that it was going to work. The miscarriage definitely cast a pall over that next pregnancy – I didn't have the same unqualified joy and freedom to think about all we'd planned. There was a lot more uncertainty, and firsthand knowledge that things could go wrong.

Of course, it didn't affect me once my daughter was born. And when I got pregnant the next time, with our son, I told everyone right away.

I don't really think about the child I might have had, because of the two children I do have. I was surprised how hard it hit me at the time, but wouldn't change anything that happened before because then my kids wouldn't be exactly who they are, and I wouldn't swap that for anything.

miscarriage management

A miscarriage will generally begin of its own accord some time after the fetus actually dies. This can happen promptly, or it can be delayed for some time. Sometimes the body retains the fetus, placenta, and other products of conception for weeks (called a "missed miscarriage" or "missed abortion"), although pregnancy symptoms disappear.

How can there be such a thing as a "missed miscarriage?" When my doctor diagnosed my first I remember thinking the idea was absurd – that it was like a "missed rainstorm" – either it happened or it didn't. How could it not happen (i.e. be "missed") but somehow still have happened?

The confusion arises because "miscarriage" refers to the failure of a pregnancy before 20 weeks' gestation. This is almost always followed by the body's expulsion of the failed pregnancy, which has come to be called a "miscarriage" as well. So while most of us think that "miscarriage" refers to the actual expulsion of the pregnancy (blood flow, tissue, etc), it refers more precisely to the actual failure of the pregnancy. Therefore, a "missed miscarriage" makes sense – it is a miscarriage (a pregnancy loss prior to 20 weeks' gestation) that has not yet been expelled by the body.

A miscarriage (i.e. a failed pregnancy) can be discovered by any of several methods, including ultrasound, blood test, pelvic exam, etc. A confirmation should be made by ultrasound scan, which will almost always give a clear answer, before any definitive action is taken. An inevitable miscarriage that has not yet begun on its own is generally treated with a "dilation and curettage," or "D&C." In this procedure, performed under general anesthetic, the cervix is dilated and a curette (suction hose) is inserted into the uterus to empty it.

A D&C ensures no products of conception remain in the uterus that could lead to infection, and for this reason D&Cs are usually performed as promptly as possible. In the past, doctors routinely recommended D&C for miscarriages at more than eight weeks gestation, even for women who spontaneously miscarried, in order to ensure no pregnancy material remained in the womb that might lead to infection. However, recently doctors have begun to argue the merits of allowing the miscarriage to proceed on its own, without any medical intervention. While this may sound more natural, and therefore preferable, D&C is associated with lower infection rates. And while infection is not common, it can be serious if it does occur, and can result in significant permanent problems such as infertility.

For women who have had an incomplete miscarriage, the great majority will go on to have a full natural miscarriage. Women with a missed miscarriage, however, are better candidates for D&C.

In any case where a D&C is optional, you will have to weigh its disadvantages against its advantages. Drawbacks include that it is a surgical end to pregnancy and an invasive procedure with some risk of after-effects. On the other hand, D&C is associated with somewhat lower risk of infection and much better chance of successful chromosomal analysis of the pregnancy tissue.

When a miscarriage happens – possible outcomes

If a miscarriage does occur, there are a variety of possible outcomes. It is important to remember that "abortion" is the medical term for an interrupted pregnancy prior to 20 weeks gestation. The word is not intended to be offensive, though it is. (I think most women would be grateful if medical professionals would use the word "miscarriage" rather than the medical term "abortion" – a word widely associated with the intentional termination of a pregnancy – when speaking to a patient who has just suffered a pregnancy loss.) Below is a summary of potential outcomes and their associated medical terms:

Threatened miscarriage (or abortion). Excessive bleeding and cramping within the first 20 weeks of pregnancy, indicating that a miscarriage may be happening.

Spontaneous miscarriage (or abortion). Natural expulsion of some or all of the products of conception.

Complete miscarriage (or abortion). Complete expulsion of all products of conception.

Incomplete miscarriage (or abortion). Incomplete expulsion of products of conception – some of the pregnancy tissue (typically the placenta) remains in the womb. Though it is usually expelled over time, it is associated with an increased risk of infection, and may need to be removed.

Inevitable miscarriage (or abortion). Miscarriage is imminent and the pregnancy cannot be saved. For example, when bleeding and pain are accompanied by rupture of the amniotic sac or dilation of the cervix.

Missed miscarriage (or abortion). The pregnancy has died (or never developed), but the body has not expelled the pregnancy materials.

Infected miscarriage (or abortion). An internal infection that can have serious consequences. Also called a "septic abortion,"

If you miscarry: miscarriage management

In the event you do miscarry, it can be difficult simply to get through what is happening. However, whatever you can learn about why the pregnancy failed can prove extremely valuable, not only for your own peace of mind, but to increase your chance of future successful pregnancies. The best information about a failed pregnancy comes from the pregnancy itself at the time of miscarriage – it is an opportunity that is very brief. So although this is a most difficult time, if tissue from the pregnancy can be collected and analyzed, answers might be found. While right now you may be unconvinced it is important or worthwhile, you are likely to find later that answers are extremely valuable.

Information you can get from a miscarriage

Without specific information to the contrary, your doctor will assume your miscarriage was due to a random chromosomal error. While this is very likely the case, you can not be fully confident without proof.

Determining the miscarried pregnancy's chromosomal profile is only possible by analysis of miscarried tissue. Unfortunately, this is not always possible, as the tissue must contain live cells. Surprisingly, the placenta can survive long after the fetus has died, so there are often live cells to analyze. However, this analysis is far more successful if tissue is collected via D&C, as with spontaneous miscarriages it has generally been dead for some time by the time it passes out of the body, and is likely contaminated. Nonetheless, if possible it is still worth collecting the tissue in a sterile container and taking it immediately to a lab for chromosomal analysis.

Whether you have a D&C or a spontaneous miscarriage, you should ensure analysis is done on any pregnancy tissue in order to determine whether there was a random chromosomal abnormality – a procedure called karyotyping. If possible, a sample of the uterine lining where it implanted should also be evaluated. Tests of these two samples can help provide the key to what went wrong in the pregnancy.

Note that a typical tissue analysis only evaluates whether the miscarriage was complete – i.e. that all tissue is accounted for. This analysis sheds no light on the possible cause of miscarriage; *you must clearly request that chromosomal analysis (karyotyping) be done if that is what you want.* I recommend that you insist, if necessary; my doctor declined to analyze my first two D&Cs, so we missed two opportunities to see that the problem lay with me, not with them.

A new system of karyotyping, called "comparative genomic hybridization" provides more accurate chromosomal analysis than the old method. In one study it accurately karyotyped 98% of tissue samples; in the remaining 2% there was not enough tissue. Traditional karyotyping gave accurate results in only 85% of cases, with 11% having inadequate tissue (the old test requires more sample than the new one), and 4% of cases returning an inaccurate karyotype. If you can get your analysis done by a lab or pathologist that uses comparative genomic hybridization, you have a much better chance of getting an accurate result.

Finally, request that the pathologist try to identify the gestational age at which the pregnancy failed. If the chromosomal analysis comes back normal, this information can be extremely valuable in pinpointing a possible cause.

If you do find that your pregnancy was chromosomally flawed then it may be some small comfort to know that miscarriages eliminate about 95% of embryos with genetic problems; most of these miscarriages are early in the pregnancy. As will be discussed in more detail later in the book, most chromosomal problems happen by chance, have nothing to do with the parents, and are unlikely to recur.

Particularly if you have had a previous loss or losses, the information that fetal karyotyping can give you becomes increasingly important. With each subsequent loss the chances that it is a recurrent maternal problem increase; proof that the loss was due to an abnormality of chromosomes or structural malformations indicates a better chance of successful pregnancy the next time, while proof that it was normal indicates that maternal causes should be investigated.

Even if analysis does not yield conclusive results, the slides are usually stored for years. At the rate at which diagnostic advances are being made, you may one day get an explanation for your loss.

After a miscarriage: where to from here?

A miscarriage is, by its nature, a life-changing event. From the moment a woman knows she is pregnant, she wonders how that pregnancy will change her life – she imagines the future with that child. *How will this impact my work? What changes will need to be made to the house? And what sort of mother will I be? Will he and I spend lazy days making sandcastles on the beach? Will she look like me? How will I be able to parent effectively when he swings the cat around by the tail, when all I really want to do is laugh? Will I help her learn to ride a bike? What will his smile look like? How will I feel on her first day of school?* That unborn child can turn out to be anything, and because of that it is a dream of the future. When that dream is shattered, we don't just lose a few weeks or months of pregnancy; we don't even just lose a "fetus" or a "baby." It is as though we lose a whole lifetime – the lifetime we were going to share with that child. We didn't mean for the idea to take on such huge proportions, but it did because we are human, and as humans we think about the future, and we wonder.

Like any traumatic event, there is no "right way" to deal with a pregnancy loss. Some women will grieve as intensely as they would the loss of a full-term birth. Others will feel they are doing okay. Some women will react by resolving to take life less for granted. Others may harbor a lingering distrust of their own bodies. Some women may want to take a long time to grieve. Others may want to put the experience behind them by redoubling the pace of their lives.

Whatever your unique needs and circumstances, there are many, many resources available to help you through this difficult time. There are support groups (in person or on-line), websites, books, counselors, friends, and family who can be called upon. We all know that the best patients – and those who recover the most quickly and completely from any ailment – are those who seek and receive appropriate treatment. This is your time to focus on healing your body, mind, and spirit through whatever means work best for you. (See *The Power of Love* for more about support.)

Looking forward

Many women who experience a miscarriage feel a powerlessness stemming from the fact that they couldn't control what was happening inside their own bodies. This feeling is often exacerbated by the good, but often misplaced, intentions of doctors or others who take charge of the miscarriage – or dismiss it – in an attempt to spare the woman further distress.

For many women, therefore, regaining control of their lives is a first step in moving on from what has happened. The rest of this book aims to address this part of the process. It will look only to the future, deconstructing miscarriage to enable you to better assess your own miscarriage risk and improve your outlook.

assessing your own risk of miscarriage

evaluate your risk

Catherine's story

I had a miscarriage – an early one. The kind that people seem to shrug off as perfectly normal. But it didn't feel normal to me. I was young and really healthy – I'd never had any kind of medical issue before, and didn't even have a regular doctor – so it had never even occurred to me that I might have any problem in pregnancy.

The doctor I went to assured me it was "just a miscarriage," smiling in that sympathetic, good-bedside-manner kind of way. She said, "They're so common. It's nothing to worry about." But I thought that at 27 years old I was way too young for it to be "just a miscarriage."

It seemed to me that there might be more to it. I wanted to know exactly why my pregnancy had miscarried. Was there something wrong with me that would make me miscarry again? Or was it really as the doctor had said, and next time it would be fine?

For me, it helps me handle a situation if I feel like I understand it. I like to have lots of information about things like this, because if I understand it, then maybe I can do something differently next time that will give me a better chance. But with my miscarriage there was no information. There was no test of anything – not of me, or the pregnancy, or even a question about family history – there was nothing at all to indicate that it wouldn't happen again.

The only thing I was sure of was that I didn't want to have another miscarriage again, ever.

After stewing for a while, I finally resolved to just see the doctor and get all my questions answered. As we talked, I realized she thought everything would be all right next time simply based on the fact that most women who have a miscarriage go on to have a healthy pregnancy the next time. She assumed I was among those women who would. But what if I wasn't? What if I was in the group of women who would have a problem? I know that group is small, but someone's got to be in it, and what made her so sure I wasn't?

I felt like she wasn't even considering whether there were things we could do to make sure I wouldn't miscarry again – it seemed like she wasn't going to bother worrying about it unless she had to. And the worst part of it was that even though I couldn't stop worrying about it, I felt like there was nothing I could actually do, except wait and see if she was right.

evaluate your risk

There *are* things you can do to evaluate – and try to reduce – your risk. A closer look at what causes miscarriage can help you understand and counteract any risk factors that might play a role in your own odds.

Factors linked to recurrent miscarriage

We have seen that the single most common factor causing miscarriage is simply the bad luck of random genetic error arising at conception or just thereafter. The great majority of other miscarriages are also attributable to bad luck, such as a poorly implanted blastocyst (fertilized egg), an improperly developed placenta, or an abnormal umbilical cord.

But while there is always a chance of miscarriage due to random bad luck, no one wants any additional risk. To assess whether we may be at greater risk of miscarriage requires determining whether we might have any of the conditions that cause *recurrent* miscarriage. Women with these underlying conditions will have lower odds of a healthy pregnancy until they are successfully treated.

The conditions that contribute to recurrent miscarriage are illustrated on the chart below, and are primarily chromosomal problems, immunological disorders, anatomical abnormalities, and hormonal imbalance. This chart differs from the one in the chapter *Miscarriage Explained* because it shows disorders responsible for *recurrent* miscarriage (rather than sporadic miscarriage caused by bad luck), and thus excludes random chance insofar as possible. Note that while random chromosomal error is typically grouped into sporadic miscarriage, the issue of advanced maternal age is a condition that affects the odds for every pregnancy, so these recurrent losses are included here. Finally, while diagnostic advances continue to reduce the number of cases for which no cause can be found, there remains a significant portion that cannot yet be explained.

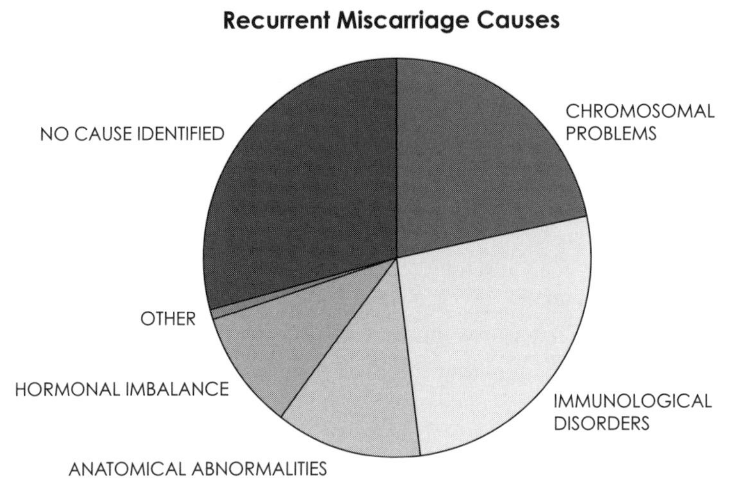

Assessing your own risk

It is important to remember that while miscarriage is very common, affecting about one in every five pregnancies, *recurrent* miscarriage is very rare – only about 1% of women will experience three or more miscarriages in a row. Thus, out of 1,000 women who become pregnant, only about 10 of those women will have three or more miscarriages. And of those 10 women, about half will have no underlying condition that makes them more prone to miscarriage – all three of their miscarriages would have been due to random chance. The other five women, however, will have an underlying condition that reduces their odds of successful pregnancy.

The next chapters are designed to help you assess whether you may be at higher risk of miscarriage. Hopefully you will find that you are one of the 995 women out of 1,000 who does not have an underlying condition. If, on the other hand, you do suspect a problem, the following chapters will give you the information you need to improve your odds.

learning from your miscarriage history

My (second) story

My miscarriages followed a specific pattern: at seven weeks there would be a good heartbeat and an embryo measuring seven weeks. But by eight weeks it would measure only seven weeks, five days, so while it had grown, it was not thriving. Much as I agonized, willing it to grow, at nine weeks it would measure eight weeks and only a couple of days. I came to know all too well what would happen next, even though I could do nothing to influence the awful course of events: by the 10th or 11th week the baby would be dead.

Although my doctor kept telling me I just had the worst luck in the world, I knew in my heart that he must be wrong.

Pregnant again after five losses, with an ultrasound at seven weeks showing a baby that looked one day too small for dates, I threw myself with renewed urgency into researching that last, most complicated cause of pregnancy loss: immunological disorders. And that was when I discovered "fetal wasting" (where the baby essentially starves because blood clots block the supply of adequate nourishment). I was sure that what I had been agonizing over on those weekly ultrasounds was fetal wasting. The treatment for this problem is simple and effective; low-dose aspirin and heparin: "blood thinners" considered safe for mother and baby.

Research also informed me that only about 3-5% of pregnancies are lost after heartbeat is confirmed; the chance of having five of those losses due to random chance is therefore only about one in ten million. My miscarriage history was clearly not just "bad luck."

It was evening, and I went immediately to buy low-dose aspirin; I took one before leaving the store.

The next morning I met with my doctor, armed with a copy of the research from a respected medical journal. He took the article and slipped it into my file without looking at it. "The aspirin won't do any good," he shrugged, "because you don't need it. But I suppose it won't do any harm either." Because he refused to believe my case was anything other than bad luck, he refused the heparin.

I rejoiced the following week when the ultrasound showed the baby was the right size. It continued to grow well until a nuchal translucency at 12 weeks showed an unrelated problem. Genetic testing confirmed the pregnancy was our only one with a chromosomal abnormality; despite the baby growing well to that point, it had a condition "not compatible with life." (In that particular case my doctor was finally right – I did have the worst luck in the world. However, firing him for all his previous ineptitude made me feel somewhat better.)

While that loss (of the pregnancy, not the doctor) was terrible, there were some significant positives that came out of it: I had taken control of my healthcare to identify, understand, and address the cause of my losses; I replaced my doctor with one who treated my concerns with respect; and I was optimistic that my next pregnancy had a good chance of success. As it happened, that next pregnancy – my last – was trouble free from conception to delivery (with my doctor's support, I began low-dose aspirin prior to conception and continued throughout the pregnancy).

The point of this story is not to encourage self-medicating, as that can actually increase the risk to you and your baby. Nor is it to encourage firing doctors who tell you things you don't want to hear (though that can be quite gratifying). The point of the story is that the explanations my doctor gave seemed hollow and wrong to me, while what I found in the research resonated with me.

My advice is to do as much research as you can, understand your options, and then make your own decisions and go with them, partnering with the very best medical professionals you can find. While the experts often disagree on how or why things work in reproductive medicine, you are completely within your rights to decide what resonates with you – what you want to try, and in whom you want to place your trust.

learning from your miscarriage history

One of the hardest things about my own miscarriages was that there was never any explanation for what might have caused them. I found it hard to move forward when the past was just a tangle of loose ends and unanswered questions.

Despite my background in medical research, and my strong interest in understanding what might be causing my losses, the only explanation my doctor would offer was "bad luck" (escalating to "very bad luck" after several losses).

When I had my first miscarriages I already knew that the most common cause of loss was random chromosomal abnormality. But I also knew this did not explain my own losses, which were tested and confirmed normal. I (as yet) knew nothing of the other problems that cause recurrent loss: immunological disorders, hormonal imbalance, and anatomical abnormalities. I didn't even know where to begin looking.

At the time, I wished for a chart like those on the following pages. I wanted something that could help me identify possible answers, and give me a head start in pinpointing the areas relevant to my own experience.

Thus, the charts on the following pages are designed to help you understand what might have caused any previous loss (or losses). Having an idea of possible causes will enable you to focus on the information most relevant to you in the chapters that follow.

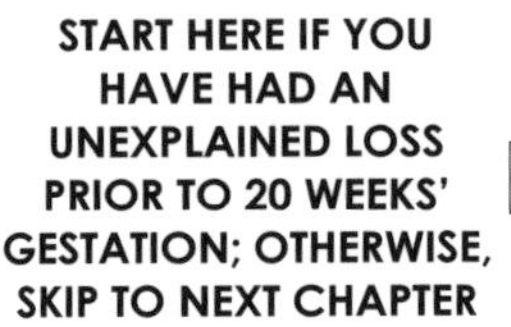

START HERE IF YOU HAVE HAD AN UNEXPLAINED LOSS PRIOR TO 20 WEEKS' GESTATION; OTHERWISE, SKIP TO NEXT CHAPTER

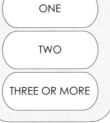

HOW MANY UNEXPLAINED MISCARRIAGES HAVE YOU HAD?

ONE

TWO

THREE OR MORE

GO TO NEXT CHART

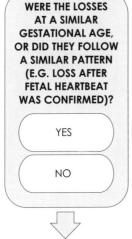

WERE THE LOSSES AT A SIMILAR GESTATIONAL AGE, OR DID THEY FOLLOW A SIMILAR PATTERN (E.G. LOSS AFTER FETAL HEARTBEAT WAS CONFIRMED)?

YES

NO

ASSESSMENT
Assess the losses as one, discounting somewhat the chance that the losses could be due to random complication

ASSESSMENT
Assess each loss separately on the following charts

WERE SOME OR ALL OF THE LOSSES AT A SIMILAR GESTATIONAL AGE, OR DID THEY FOLLOW A SIMILAR PATTERN (E.G. LOSS AFTER FETAL HEARTBEAT WAS CONFIRMED)?

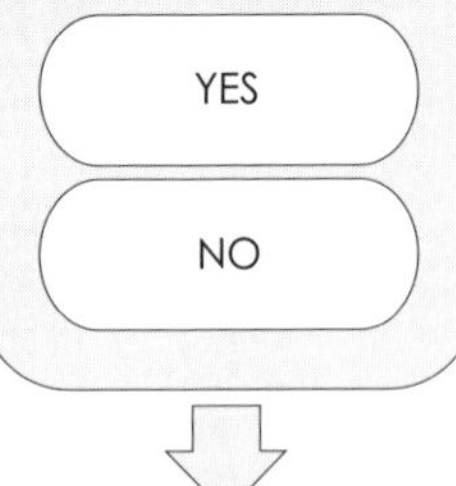

YES

NO

ASSESSMENT
The likelihood that your miscarriages were due to random chance decreases as the number of miscarriages increases. Your losses are more likely due to an underlying condition, rather than random chance.

Assess similar losses as one, discounting that they could be due to random chance.

ASSESSMENT
The likelihood that your miscarriages were due to random chance decreases as the number of miscarriages increases.

Assess each loss separately on the following charts to determine if any pattern emerges.

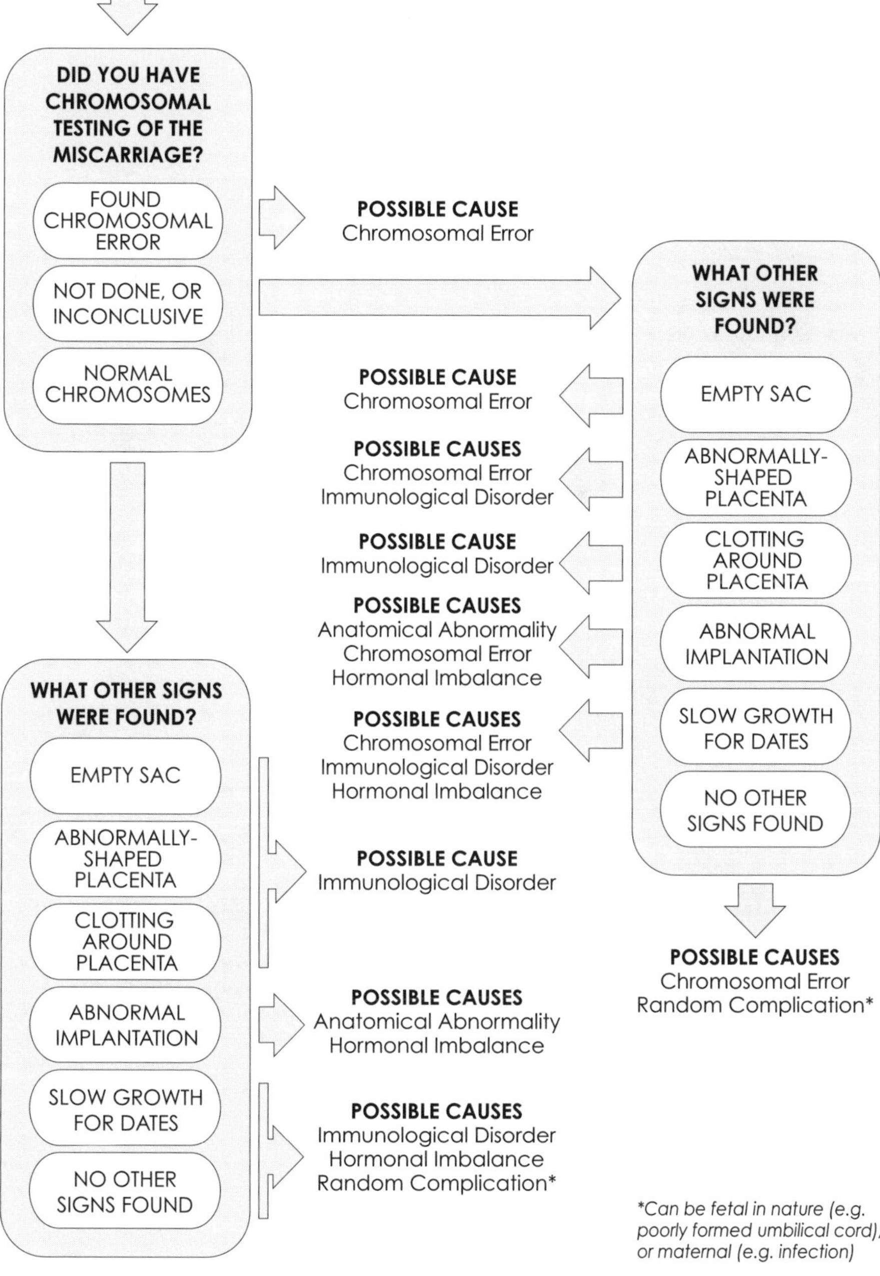
START HERE IF YOUR MISCARRIAGE OCCURRED
BY 8 WEEKS; OTHERWISE, SKIP TO THE NEXT CHART
DID YOU HAVE CHROMOSOMAL TESTING OF THE MISCARRIAGE?
FOUND CHROMOSOMAL ERROR
NOT DONE, OR INCONCLUSIVE
NORMAL CHROMOSOMES
POSSIBLE CAUSE
Chromosomal Error
WHAT OTHER SIGNS WERE FOUND?
EMPTY SAC
ABNORMALLY-SHAPED PLACENTA
CLOTTING AROUND PLACENTA
ABNORMAL IMPLANTATION
SLOW GROWTH FOR DATES
NO OTHER SIGNS FOUND
POSSIBLE CAUSE
Chromosomal Error
POSSIBLE CAUSES
Chromosomal Error
Immunological Disorder
POSSIBLE CAUSE
Immunological Disorder
POSSIBLE CAUSES
Anatomical Abnormality
Chromosomal Error
Hormonal Imbalance
POSSIBLE CAUSES
Chromosomal Error
Immunological Disorder
Hormonal Imbalance
POSSIBLE CAUSES
Chromosomal Error
Random Complication*
WHAT OTHER SIGNS WERE FOUND?
EMPTY SAC
ABNORMALLY-SHAPED PLACENTA
CLOTTING AROUND PLACENTA
ABNORMAL IMPLANTATION
SLOW GROWTH FOR DATES
NO OTHER SIGNS FOUND
POSSIBLE CAUSE
Immunological Disorder
POSSIBLE CAUSES
Anatomical Abnormality
Hormonal Imbalance
POSSIBLE CAUSES
Immunological Disorder
Hormonal Imbalance
Random Complication*
*Can be fetal in nature (e.g. poorly formed umbilical cord), or maternal (e.g. infection)

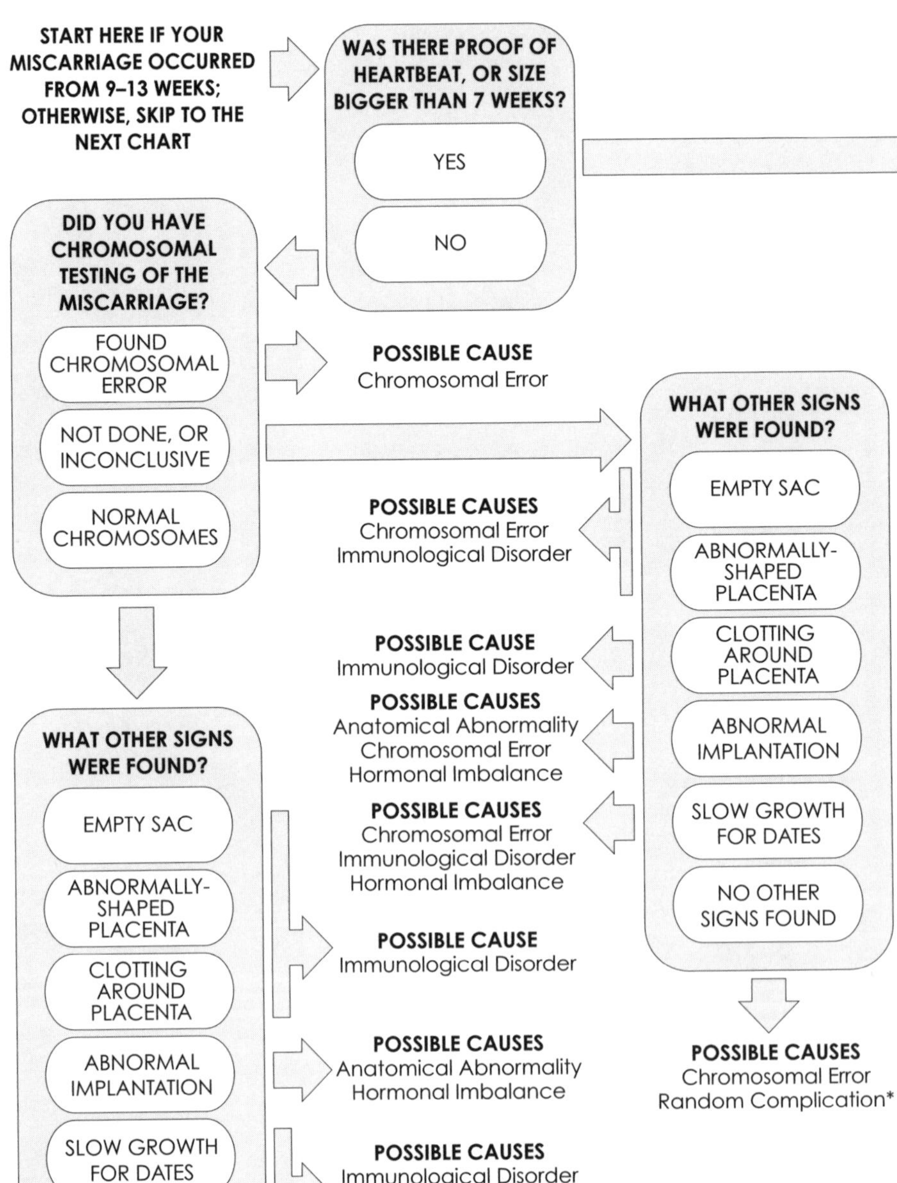
START HERE IF YOUR MISCARRIAGE OCCURRED FROM 9–13 WEEKS; OTHERWISE, SKIP TO THE NEXT CHART
WAS THERE PROOF OF HEARTBEAT, OR SIZE BIGGER THAN 7 WEEKS?
YES
NO
DID YOU HAVE CHROMOSOMAL TESTING OF THE MISCARRIAGE?
FOUND CHROMOSOMAL ERROR
NOT DONE, OR INCONCLUSIVE
NORMAL CHROMOSOMES
POSSIBLE CAUSE
Chromosomal Error
WHAT OTHER SIGNS WERE FOUND?
EMPTY SAC
ABNORMALLY-SHAPED PLACENTA
CLOTTING AROUND PLACENTA
ABNORMAL IMPLANTATION
SLOW GROWTH FOR DATES
NO OTHER SIGNS FOUND
POSSIBLE CAUSES
Chromosomal Error
Immunological Disorder
POSSIBLE CAUSE
Immunological Disorder
POSSIBLE CAUSES
Anatomical Abnormality
Chromosomal Error
Hormonal Imbalance
POSSIBLE CAUSES
Chromosomal Error
Immunological Disorder
Hormonal Imbalance
POSSIBLE CAUSES
Chromosomal Error
Random Complication*
WHAT OTHER SIGNS WERE FOUND?
EMPTY SAC
ABNORMALLY-SHAPED PLACENTA
CLOTTING AROUND PLACENTA
ABNORMAL IMPLANTATION
SLOW GROWTH FOR DATES
NO OTHER SIGNS FOUND
POSSIBLE CAUSE
Immunological Disorder
POSSIBLE CAUSES
Anatomical Abnormality
Hormonal Imbalance
POSSIBLE CAUSES
Immunological Disorder
Random Complication*
Hormonal Imbalance

DID YOU HAVE CHROMOSOMAL TESTING OF THE MISCARRIAGE?

- FOUND CHROMOSOMAL ERROR → **POSSIBLE CAUSE** Chromosomal Error
- NOT DONE, OR INCONCLUSIVE → WHAT OTHER SIGNS WERE FOUND?
- NORMAL CHROMOSOMES → WHAT OTHER SIGNS WERE FOUND?

WHAT OTHER SIGNS WERE FOUND? (not done, or inconclusive)

- ABNORMALLY-SHAPED PLACENTA → **POSSIBLE CAUSES** Chromosomal Error, Immunological Disorder
- CLOTTING AROUND PLACENTA → **POSSIBLE CAUSE** Immunological Disorder
- ABNORMAL IMPLANTATION → **POSSIBLE CAUSES** Anatomical Abnormality, Chromosomal Error
- SLOW GROWTH FOR DATES → **POSSIBLE CAUSES** Chromosomal Error, Immunological Disorder
- NO OTHER SIGNS FOUND → **POSSIBLE CAUSES** Chromosomal Error, Immunological Disorder, Anatomical Abnormality, Random Complication*

WHAT OTHER SIGNS WERE FOUND? (normal chromosomes)

- ABNORMALLY-SHAPED PLACENTA, CLOTTING AROUND PLACENTA → **POSSIBLE CAUSE** Immunological Disorder
- ABNORMAL IMPLANTATION → **POSSIBLE CAUSE** Anatomical Abnormality
- SLOW GROWTH FOR DATES, NO OTHER SIGNS FOUND → **POSSIBLE CAUSES** Immunological Disorder, Anatomical Abnormality, Random Complication*

**Can be fetal in nature (e.g. poorly formed umbilical cord), or maternal (e.g. infection)*

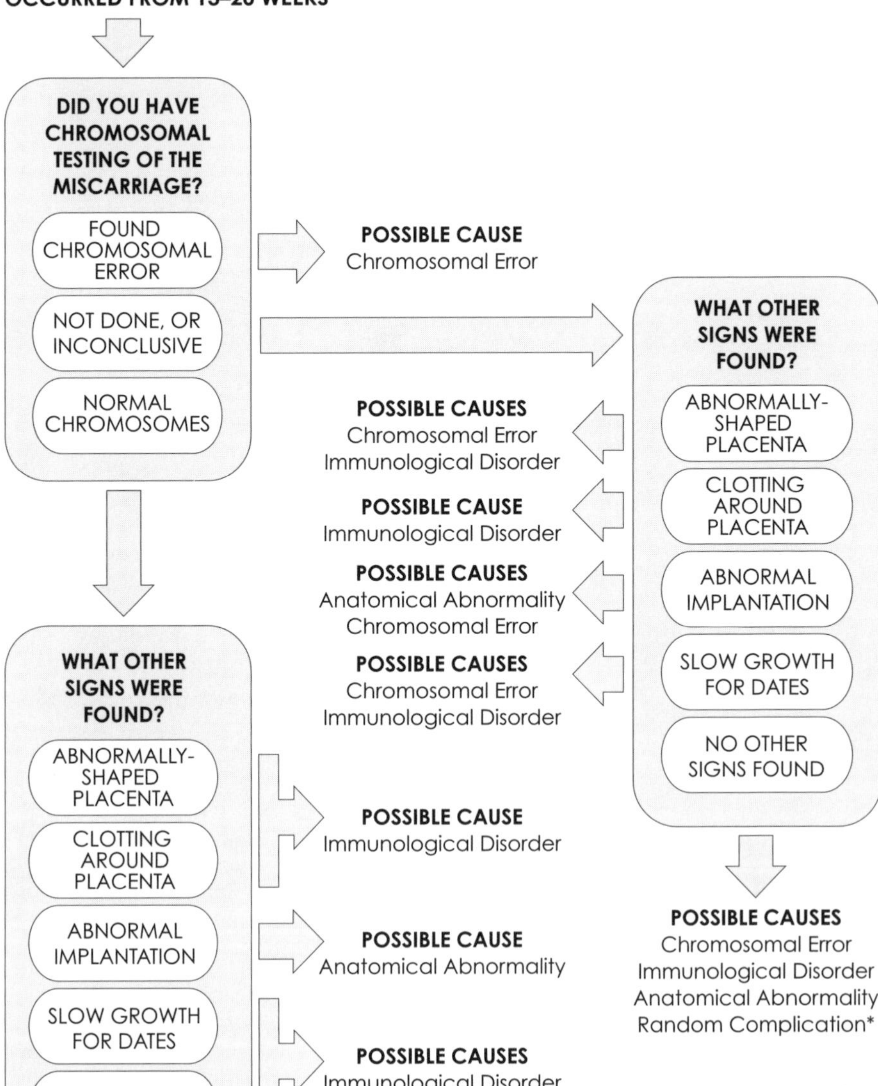
START HERE IF YOUR MISCARRIAGE OCCURRED FROM 13–20 WEEKS
DID YOU HAVE CHROMOSOMAL TESTING OF THE MISCARRIAGE?
FOUND CHROMOSOMAL ERROR
NOT DONE, OR INCONCLUSIVE
NORMAL CHROMOSOMES
POSSIBLE CAUSE
Chromosomal Error
WHAT OTHER SIGNS WERE FOUND?
ABNORMALLY-SHAPED PLACENTA
CLOTTING AROUND PLACENTA
ABNORMAL IMPLANTATION
SLOW GROWTH FOR DATES
NO OTHER SIGNS FOUND
POSSIBLE CAUSES
Chromosomal Error
Immunological Disorder
POSSIBLE CAUSE
Immunological Disorder
POSSIBLE CAUSES
Anatomical Abnormality
Chromosomal Error
POSSIBLE CAUSES
Chromosomal Error
Immunological Disorder
POSSIBLE CAUSES
Chromosomal Error
Immunological Disorder
Anatomical Abnormality
Random Complication*
WHAT OTHER SIGNS WERE FOUND?
ABNORMALLY-SHAPED PLACENTA
CLOTTING AROUND PLACENTA
ABNORMAL IMPLANTATION
SLOW GROWTH FOR DATES
NO OTHER SIGNS FOUND
POSSIBLE CAUSE
Immunological Disorder
POSSIBLE CAUSE
Anatomical Abnormality
POSSIBLE CAUSES
Immunological Disorder
Anatomical Abnormality
Random Complication*
*Can be fetal in nature (e.g. poorly formed umbilical cord) or maternal (e.g. infection)

A testing option if you have miscarried previously

If you have miscarried previously and had a D&C when you lost your pregnancy (or brought tissue in to be analyzed after a spontaneous miscarriage), then it is likely that the tissue exists in paraffin blocks in the pathology department of the hospital where the procedure was performed. (Tissue is encased in paraffin – a special kind of wax – in order to allow sectioning and analysis of the sample.) Experts claim that these are retained for decades.

Some specialist centers now offer testing on these blocks, claiming that they can assess a variety of factors including placental attachment, immunological disorders, evidence of chromosomal abnormality, and gestational age. If so, this analysis could eliminate or focus the tests necessary to diagnose underlying maternal problems.

Summary

While it can be distressing to analyze previous losses, the analysis can help illuminate the way forward by pinpointing areas that may be of interest to you.

Each of the following chapters will include detailed explanation and a self-assessment questionnaire to help you evaluate areas of interest, and determine whether you may be at higher risk for any of the disorders that cause recurrent miscarriage. Less common causes such as maternal disease and environmental exposures are covered in the last chapter of this section.

By the end of this part of the book you will have evaluated your own miscarriage risk profile. If you find you are not at greater risk of an underlying condition, then that information should provide comfort. If, on the other hand, you find you may be at increased risk, then you will have the information you need to improve your own miscarriage outlook.

chromosomal problems

Jill's story

I had always wanted three or four kids. I was 36 when we started trying to get pregnant, and it happened quickly and easily – we were pregnant with Jean-Christophe within two months. When we tried for our second child it took longer – it was nine months before I got pregnant with Alexandra. Still, I never thought the clock was ticking, or that there might be a problem.

After that I had three miscarriages over two years. All three tested genetically abnormal.

By then I was 41, and we went to a fertility specialist. From there we decided to do IVF, and over the next two years we did four full rounds.

I found the whole process of IVF emotionally and physically painful, and think it wreaks havoc on a marriage. Everything you do is timed! For weeks I was giving myself four shots a day, and had to be in the clinic every morning by 6.30 to have a blood test to recalibrate my medication. And it's a production line – there are 20 other women in there doing exactly the same thing.

Every day you're on pins and needles, fearing that your nurse will call you and tell you it's not worth continuing – that not enough follicles are ripening for the harvesting to be worthwhile.

Harvesting itself is done under general anesthetic, and once you wake up all you want to know is how many eggs they got. It's demoralizing. There are curtains around you, but everyone can hear everything. The doctor told me we got only eight eggs; I heard them tell the woman next to me that she got 40, or some huge amount.

Then you're waiting for the call about how fertilization went. Are they growing? Do they look viable? Healthy?

You go back to the clinic three days later and they transfer some embryos to your womb while you watch on an ultrasound. Then it's progesterone shots for two weeks until you find out if you're pregnant. After all those weeks of shots your arms, hips, and abdomen are killing you. Your veins ache.

And then you're waiting for another call – though it's 10-12 days away – telling you if you're pregnant.

Out of four full rounds of IVF we got only one pregnancy, which miscarried. Though it had been visually assessed, it turned out to have a chromosomal problem. My clinic didn't offer PGD [preimplantation genetic diagnosis, discussed later in this chapter].

IVF is physically painful, but emotionally it's even worse – you're wound up like a clock. A woman should know this going in and get her support group firmly in place.

They tell you before you start IVF that you should have an end in mind – how long you'll go until you stop. I didn't, but after the fourth round I knew that was it. I couldn't take anymore. At that stage I realized we were not going to have another child.

You hear about actresses or famous people having kids really late, so you think, "Why can't I do that?" My doctor says a lot of those women use donor eggs. They make it seem more possible than it is.

Now, when friends are cavalier about putting off having kids, I tell them what happened to me. It took me a long time to get the "Aha!" realization that the Biological Clock could (and did) happen to me. For anyone out there who cares to listen, all I can say is "Don't delay, don't delay, don't delay!"

chromosomal problems

So what if you *have* delayed? Or what if you *must* delay?

While having children at 25 may be biologically ideal, for many women it is an unattainably or undesirably early deadline. Whether because it takes longer to find the right life partner, or to achieve the right life balance, or for a million other reasons, many women are starting their families later. And so, for women looking at delaying childbearing to their 30s and beyond, it is necessary to understand the risks and choices of later motherhood.

As we have seen, chromosomal abnormality is the most common cause of sporadic miscarriage, accounting for more than half of those losses. But what role does chromosomal abnormality play in recurrent miscarriage?

Unless one of the partners is carrying a genetic abnormality, chromosomal problems are traditionally grouped into the statistics for sporadic miscarriage. But for older women the problem of poor egg quality is a recurrent one that affects the odds for every pregnancy, as it is due to the underlying condition of having older eggs. When these miscarriages are included in the statistics for recurrent miscarriage causes, chromosomal problems account for about 20-25% of all recurrent losses.

Although losses due to chromosomal problems can occur throughout pregnancy, the abnormalities themselves are present at the moment of conception, or very shortly thereafter.

As previously discussed, every cell in the human body – with the exception of the egg and sperm cells – contains 46 chromosomes: 23

matched pairs. While chromosomes look surprisingly unimpressive – like thick, floppy pieces of yarn – they contain all our genes. Genes instruct cellular performance essential to healthy bodily function. Scientists estimate that there are 25,000-75,000 human genes, which means each chromosome contains hundreds or thousands of them. (I imagine chromosomes as bookshelves stuffed with hundreds or thousands of books, which are the genes.)

Abnormalities can involve the chromosomes themselves, or just one or more genes. Most gene abnormalities do not result in an abnormality in the embryo unless the faulty gene is inherited from both the mother and the father; if only one copy of the gene is defective, then the normal gene from the other parent will usually take over.

Chromosomal problems, however, are far more serious, as they involve many genes. Errors arise when the chromosomes do not do exactly what they're supposed to do, or go exactly where they're supposed to go. Pieces of chromosome can break off and reattach in a different order, interchange with other chromosomes, be copied more than once, or be lost completely. When these mistakes occur early in the reproductive process, they typically lead to miscarriage.

Many chromosomal abnormalities arise simply from the imperfect execution of a highly complex process – they are sporadic (random), and nothing can be done to predict or anticipate these chance errors. What we are concerned with here, therefore, are conditions that result in a higher proportion of flawed embryos – i.e. underlying, permanent problems that increase the likelihood of miscarriage due to chromosomal abnormality.

It is important to remember that chromosomal abnormalities cannot be controlled – they are nobody's fault. But that is not to say that nothing can be done to combat genetic problems that are likely to recur – there *are* ways of evaluating and addressing these risks.

Self-assessment

As has been described, chromosomal abnormalities can be introduced via the eggs, sperm, or both. Thus, the following questionnaire is for both you and your partner, and is designed to help each of you assess whether you might be at higher risk of genetic problems.

Self-assessment: chromosomal problems

(Tick the box for Yes)

	You	Partner
1. *Do you have family* with chromosomal or genetic abnormality (e.g. Down's syndrome, cystic fibrosis)?*	☐	☐
2. *Do you have family* with retardation, physical or mental abnormalities?*	☐	☐
3. *Are you descended from any coupling of close relatives, or related to your partner?*	☐	☐
4. *Do you have family* with recurrent miscarriage that could be genetic in nature?*	☐	☐
5. *Have you had a pregnancy with a genetic defect?*	☐	
6. *Have you had two or more first trimester pregnancy losses that may have been genetically abnormal?*	☐	
7. *Are you over 35 (women), or 40 (men)?*	☐	☐
8. *Have you been exposed to serious environmental toxins (e.g. radiation)?*	☐	☐
9. *Did your mother take DES when pregnant with you?*	☐	
10. *Have you experienced infertility?*	☐	☐

Interpreting the results

If you and your partner answered No to each of these questions

There is no reason to think you are at greater risk of having a genetically abnormal embryo, and you should skip to the next self-assessment chapter, *Immunological Disorders*.

---

* Grandparents, parents, siblings, aunts, uncles, or first cousins directly related to you by blood, not marriage (i.e. descended from a common ancestor).

If you or your partner answered Yes to any of questions 1-6

You may be at a higher risk of maternal or paternal genetic disorder – i.e. an error in your own chromosomes that you pass on. Luckily, this is an unusual condition, and testing is straightforward. Reading the section "Maternal or Paternal Genetic Disorder," below, should help you better understand how to evaluate and address any risk you might have.

If you or your partner answered Yes to any of questions 5-10

You may have poor egg or sperm quality, or a higher likelihood of failure in the fertilization or replication processes. Reading the sections "Defective Cellular Function" and "Problems in Fertilization or Replication," below, should help you better understand how to evaluate and address any risk you might have.

An in-depth look at chromosomal problems

Problems of a chromosomal nature are either present in the egg or sperm prior to conception, or arise in the fertilization or replication processes. These are explained in detail below.

Problems in the egg or sperm prior to conception

Genetic abnormalities in the egg or sperm can arise from two sources discussed in detail below: an underlying maternal or paternal genetic disorder, or improper cellular function prior to fertilization.

Regardless of the cause, any genetic abnormality in the egg or sperm will be directly reflected in the blueprint set of chromosomes, and would be expected to result in miscarriage of the resultant embryo. All of these problems are treated in much the same way, and are discussed in the section "Treatment and Success Rates."

Underlying maternal or paternal genetic disorder

Couples who have miscarried often worry that they may have passed an abnormality on to their pregnancy, but this is very rarely the case (only 3-5% of couples who experience recurrent miscarriage will find it is due to a genetic problem in one of the partners). Any abnormality in the maternal or paternal genes would not usually result in a miscarriage – the parents themselves are proof of that. However, if the egg and sperm contain matching abnormalities, the combination can prove lethal. (Partners that are related to each other have a higher miscarriage rate precisely because they are more likely to have matching genetic abnormalities.)

Testing

A simple blood test will establish your "karyotype" (your unique chromosomes), which will be screened for abnormalities. This test is generally done by a genetic counselor (also called a "clinical geneticist"), who is an expert on genes and chromosomes. Geneticists can be found at fertility clinics and many medical centers, and you do not need a referral from your doctor to schedule a consultation. Results typically include an image of the 23 chromosome pairs.

If it is found that you or your partner *do* have a chromosomal abnormality, then consultation with a genetic counselor is essential. There *are* options available to you, ranging from no intervention at all (couples with the most common types of chromosomal abnormalities can have a 40-50% chance of a healthy baby following natural conception) to extensive intervention with IVF and PGD (discussed later in this chapter).

Defective cellular function

Many women are told their losses have a simple cause: "age." As discussed in the chapter *Miscarriage Explained*, age has a significant negative effect on egg cell function. Studies have shown that as women age, errors accumulate in the eggs, and division into two sets of chromosomes becomes unreliable. One study found that about seven out of every 10 eggs were irregular in women over 35 (though these irregularities included the eggs' structure and functioning, and many of these irregularities may not have led to genetic abnormality or miscarriage).

"Meiosis" is the process of separating one set of 23 paired chromosomes into two sets of 23 *unpaired* chromosomes (somewhat akin to "unzipping" the chromosomes), and is central to the formation of egg cells. Oddly, whereas sperm are created with only 23 unpaired chromosomes, egg cells have 23 *paired* sets of chromosomes until just before conception; meiosis must occur perfectly to produce a high-quality egg.

Recent studies suggest that the process of meiosis becomes increasingly error-prone with age, and in some individuals is flawed at any age, leading to the frequent retention or loss of a chromosome. If the egg or sperm has an extra copy of a chromosome, or is missing it altogether, the resultant embryo will also have the wrong number of chromosomes. "Monosomy" (only one copy of a chromosome) is the most common chromosomal abnormality causing miscarriage. An embryo with "trisomy" (three copies of a chromosome) would also be expected to miscarry. A woman's body eliminates more than 95% of chromosomally flawed pregnancies through miscarriage, with fewer than five in every 100 chromosomally abnormal fetuses surviving to birth. It is not known why some of these pregnancies survive while others don't (e.g. some trisomy-21 (Down's Syndrome) babies not only survive till birth, but live to an average age of nearly 60, according to the Down's Syndrome Association).

While research indicates that men can have genetically abnormal sperm, until recently it was thought that only a defective egg could lead to a chromosomal abnormality within the embryo that would result in miscarriage. Thus, little work has been done in this area. However, work to date suggests that environmental factors (perhaps even cigarette smoke) may produce the kinds of genetic breaks in sperm that are implicated in miscarriage.

Testing

Testing for poor egg and sperm quality requires testing the actual eggs or sperm – there is no simple blood or urine test that can give this information.

Because sperm are easy to obtain, assessing their quality is straightforward and done routinely at fertility clinics (though you must specify *chromosomal* analysis, which is not standard).

Eggs, however, are only tiny specks in the ovaries – they are difficult to access and remove, and doing so requires the preparation regime, specialist doctors, and specialized equipment associated with the IVF process. Thus, eggs are typically only assessed as part of a broader program to combat infertility or recurrent miscarriage. The details of this process are explained below, in "Treatment and Success Rates."

Problems in fertilization or replication

While fertilization sounds simple – the fusion of egg and sperm – it is actually a very complex process that must result in two sets of unpaired chromosomes combining into one set of perfectly-paired chromosomes. Chromosomes that break off, interchange, or end up in the wrong place will create a chromosomal abnormality. As with faulty eggs and sperm, any abnormality present at this early stage will compromise the blueprint set of chromosomes, and would be expected to miscarry.

If a fertilized egg has made it this far without error, it is highly likely to remain so. However, replication errors can still occur. If an error occurs early in the process, it can have a devastating effect, because the early cells give rise to all other cells. For example, even if fertilization created a perfect blueprint set of paired chromosomes, if the very first replication introduced an error, then there would be one perfect cell (the original fused cell) and one damaged cell (the improperly copied cell). These two cells would then replicate themselves, and then those cells would replicate themselves, and so on. The resulting embryo would have 50% normal cells, and 50% abnormal cells. This condition, where only a portion of the chromosomes are abnormal, is called "mosaic." While a mosaic embryo or fetus may survive longer than it would have had it been 100% abnormal, the pregnancy is still typically lost.

Testing

The success of fertilization and early replication can only be determined from actual embryos. Currently there is only one way to use chromosomal analysis to actually reduce the chance of miscarriage. This diagnosis, called preimplantation genetic diagnosis (PGD) is only performed outside the womb (i.e. on IVF embryos). It is the process by which a number of early-stage embryos are tested for chromosomal abnormalities in order to determine which should be returned to the womb. By screening for problems *before* implantation, a couple at high risk of chromosomally abnormal embryos can improve their chance of a healthy pregnancy. (Methods such as amniocentesis, that test the fetus in the womb, cannot improve the chance of a healthy pregnancy – they can only reveal the chromosomal makeup of the fetus already there.) The PGD testing process is more fully explained in "Treatment and Success Rates," below.

Molar pregnancy: a special case

Hydatidiform moles are a rare condition that occur only once in every 1,500-1,800 pregnancies. Simply called molar pregnancies, these can be caused either by a problem in the egg (complete mole) or a problem of fertilization (partial mole). An embryo either does not form at all, or is so severely malformed that it cannot survive.

Complete moles. Complete moles occur when a sperm fertilizes an egg sac lacking the maternal DNA (called an empty egg sac). There is only one of each chromosome – all paternal. Though no embryo is present, the placenta grows in a rapid, uncontrolled manner, giving the appearance of a bubbly mass.

In a small portion of cases (about 15%), the mole develops into a kind of cancer, growing rapidly and spreading to other areas of the body. If this happens then prompt specialist treatment is essential.

Partial moles. Far less severe than complete moles, partial moles occur when two sperm fertilize an egg; the resultant embryo has three copies of each chromosome. While the placenta grows rapidly, and placental cells swell with fluid, it is not to the same extent as in a complete mole, and can be missed on an ultrasound. While partial moles develop into the cancer-like form only very rarely, it is nonetheless important to get specialist care and follow-up.

Testing and treatment

A molar pregnancy begins like a regular pregnancy, but around week 10-12 there is often dark brown bleeding. Also, women with molar pregnancies tend to have HCG levels that are too high (in the case of a complete mole) or too low (in the case of a partial mole), and a uterus that is larger than normal. These conditions can lead to severe nausea and vomiting, high blood pressure, and abdominal cramps.

Often a woman with a partial molar pregnancy will have the same symptoms as a normal miscarriage, and only through chromosomal analysis of pregnancy tissue is it identified as a partial mole.

If a molar pregnancy is suspected, it should be confirmed by ultrasound and evaluation of HCG levels. If a molar is confirmed, complete removal of all molar tissue is necessary as there is a chance that molar cells can continue to grow and become cancerous. This is usually done by D&C under general anesthetic.

After removal, HCG levels must be regularly monitored to ensure they return to zero. In some cases (about 15-20% of complete moles, and less than 5% of partial moles), traces of the abnormal molar tissue continue to grow, requiring treatment with one or more cancer drugs. Because of the chance that abnormal tissue will continue to grow, women are advised not to become pregnant again for 6-12 months after removal of a mole, as the rising HCG of a pregnancy would mask signs that molar tissue is still active.

Women who have experienced a molar pregnancy have a good outlook for future success; only 1-2% will experience another mole.

If you want to find out more without testing

To find out more about chromosomal issues to help clarify your own risk profile, you can speak to a genetic counselor. While it is impossible to determine your precise risk without testing, this specialist can discuss with you your specific situation and concerns, and provide valuable assistance in helping you assess your risk of infertility and miscarriage (because if you *do* have a recurrent genetic problem, it may result in either, or both, problems).

Treatment and success rates

Medical science cannot yet repair abnormal chromosomes; if you have a genetic problem, then there is currently nothing that can be done to correct this. However, something may be able to be done to increase your chances of a genetically healthy pregnancy. But the "incurable" nature of chromosomal abnormality means it requires the most extensive medical intervention of any condition causing miscarriage. While this may not be the avenue you choose, it can be comforting to know that there *are* options for tackling this difficult problem. The information below is intended to reassure you that there are ways of combating what has traditionally been an untreatable problem. It is not the only way forward. Couples with the most common genetic abnormalities have about a 40-50% chance of normal pregnancy without intervention.

If you do not want to contemplate extensive intervention at this time, just skip the next section; if you are interested in finding out what medical science has devised to increase the odds of a healthy pregnancy for couples with chromosomal problems, read on.

Turning back the hands of time?

Recurrent chromosomal problems – regardless of their origin – are all treated in much the same way. Whether the abnormality arises from the parental genes, the eggs, the sperm, the fertilization process, or early replication, each of these problems is addressed in assisted reproductive technology (ART). ART was formerly referred to as IVF (in vitro fertilization), but encompasses many techniques and technologies, and should not be thought of as being only for infertile couples. Couples that have a significant risk of producing embryos with chromosomal disorders may benefit from these techniques, which are constantly developing and improving.

For couples prepared to invest a good deal of energy and money, many of the factors that work against older mothers – or anyone with increased genetic risk – can be assessed, addressed, and improved.

While we've all heard of IVF, most of us don't know how it might help prevent miscarriage. "In vitro" simply means "in glass," while "in vivo" means "in life," which refers to the conventional way of becoming pregnant. Essentially, IVF is the process of becoming pregnant with the assistance of the latest medical technology, using the woman's eggs and her partner's sperm. The benefit is that each step of the reproductive process is monitored and evaluated, so that you can be sure of exactly what is going on. The drawback is that each step of the reproductive process is monitored and evaluated, which many women like Jill find emotionally and physically draining. However, if the IVF process is undertaken, then only the healthiest embryos can be chosen for return to the womb, which may increase the chance of a healthy pregnancy and reduce the risk of miscarriage. The five-step process is summarized below:

Step 1. Ovarian stimulation: Medication is given for 2-4 weeks that stimulates the ovary to ripen several eggs, rather than the single egg that usually develops each month. Each egg develops in a follicle in the ovary, and follicles can be seen and assessed on an ultrasound.

Step 2. Egg retrieval: Using ultrasound, a needle is passed through the vagina into the ovary, removing the egg from each follicle. On average, about 12 eggs are retrieved. The procedure is done under sedation or anesthetic, and takes 15-30 minutes.

Step 3. Fertilization and early replication: Sperm is mixed with the eggs, and they are incubated. Eggs that are not fertilized or growing properly are discarded.

Step 4. Preimplantation genetic diagnosis (PGD): When the embryo has 6-8 cells (day 3), it can be tested for chromosomal abnormality.

Step 5. Embryo transfer: Normal embryos are implanted in the womb.

For couples who produce a greater proportion of embryos with chromosomal abnormality, PGD may reduce the chance of miscarriage by screening for them. While PGD has been used successfully for more than a decade, it is an advanced and costly technical process, and most centers do not offer it, instead offering only "embryo grading," which is not the same. Embryo grading is done by looking at embryos under a microscope and assessing their appearance. Unfortunately, up to 50% of embryos that look healthy can contain genetic abnormalities. Of the centers that do carry out PGD, some will test one cell, and some two; those that test two cells do so to provide an extra check against a mosaic embryo, in which there are both normal and abnormal cells.

Recent studies on IVF embryos have found that 40-75% have a chromosomal abnormality; the great majority of these are mosaic. In addition, most abnormal embryos appeared normal to experts who visually assessed them. Thus, as Jill found with her pregnancy that was visually assessed as normal but proved to be abnormal when miscarriage tissue was analyzed, your chance of transferring a normal embryo increases if you are at a center doing PGD, especially if the analysis is based on two cells rather than one.

Outlook

Opinions on the benefits of PGD conflict dramatically. Some centers claim great success. For example, one center reported on a group of women whose past reproductive performance had totaled 115 pregnancies which had resulted in 104 miscarriages and only 11 deliveries. The transfer of PGD-screened embryos in this group led to an 84% "take home baby rate." While many of these women probably required a number of attempts with multiple embryos, the results are nonetheless impressive.

But more recent, well-designed studies convincingly draw the conclusion that there is no significant benefit of PGD compared to regular IVF. A possible explanation is that specialists have become more skilled at visual assessment, and therefore transfer a higher proportion of healthy embryos in the regular IVF group. Or that some factor negatively impacted the success of the PGD embryos in recent studies. Or perhaps there really is no significant benefit to transferring two normal embryos compared to three visually graded embryos – it is not yet known *how* normal a 6-8 cell embryo has to be to ultimately produce a normal baby. The assumption that normal babies can only result from embryos that were 100% normal at the 6-8 cell stage has never been tested or proven, and it is possible that certain cases of mosaic abnormality might normalize. (For example, if abnormal cells replicate poorly or not at all, they could be quickly overtaken by normal cells.)

For now, PGD raises as many questions as it answers, and more work needs to be done before its benefits become completely clear.

Thus, if you are considering PGD you need to weigh several factors: PGD means going through IVF even though you may be fertile; it adds significantly to the cost of IVF; misdiagnosis or lethal damage to the embryo are real possibilities; and the benefits are still being debated. On the other hand, PGD could be of particular help to couples with known genetic abnormalities they do not want to pass on to their children.

As with any treatment, the success rates of the specialists you choose may make all the difference to the outcome. Generally, success rates for a single embryo testing normal on PGD are estimated at approximately 38% for women under 35 years old, 25% for women 35-39, and 15% for women over 40. This means that older women will need to have more than one embryo transferred to achieve the success rates seen in younger women. (For example, if 16 women aged 35-39 each had two healthy PGD embryos transferred, we would expect eight women to be unsuccessful, seven to have one child, and one woman to have twins.)

Choosing a center

American fertility clinics are required by law to report their success rates to the government, and these can be obtained from the Centers for Disease Control and Prevention (CDC) or its website. Success rates vary widely (from 12% to over 50%) depending on the center. Be aware that some centers may apply more stringent screening criteria in order to keep their success rates high. If you are interested in PGD then you must ensure in advance that the center you choose offers chromosomal testing of fertilized embryos prior to returning them to the womb (PGD), and not only visual assessment.

How to initiate treatment

IVF is considered appropriate for couples who have a history of recurrent miscarriage or infertility (at least 12 months in younger women, and six months in women over 35). You will not generally require a referral or specific medical documentation to be accepted as an IVF patient. PGD is thought to particularly benefit couples who make a high proportion of chromosomally abnormal embryos, such as couples with a genetic abnormality; its benefit to older women is still being debated. PGD is available to IVF patients for an additional fee so long as the clinic offers the procedure.

Summary

Though couples with higher risk of recurrent chromosomal problems clearly face great challenges, there *are* options. While it requires extensive medical intervention, and a great investment of energy and money, PGD may help improve the odds of achieving a normal pregnancy and delivering a healthy baby.

Testing and treatment options for the various conditions causing chromosomal abnormalities are summarized on the following page.

SUMMARY TESTS FOR CHROMOSOMAL PROBLEMS				
Problem	**Test**	**Requires**	**Results**	**Total cost**
Fetal chromosomal abnormality	Chromosomal testing of tissue	Immediate analysis of miscarried tissue by specialist lab (karyotyping)	Determines embryo's specific chromosomal profile	$400-$1,000
Maternal/paternal genetic disorder	Maternal/paternal karyotype	Blood test	Determines specific maternal/ paternal chromosomal profile	$250-$500 per person
Poor sperm quality	Test of sperm sample	Genetic analysis of sperm sample	Determines proportion of chromosomally abnormal sperm	$400-$600
Poor egg quality Faulty fertilization Replication errors	PGD	Preimplantation genetic diagnosis: only done as part of IVF process	Screens fertilized eggs for chromosomal abnormality	PGD adds $2,000- $3,000 to the cost of IVF

SUMMARY TREATMENTS FOR CHROMOSOMAL PROBLEMS				
Problem	**Treatment**	**Requires**	**Pregnancy success rates**	**Total cost**
Maternal / paternal genetic disorder Poor sperm quality Poor egg quality Faulty fertilization Replication errors	Cannot currently be reversed, but IVF with PGD can identify healthy embryos	Must be a patient of a fertility center that performs IVF and PGD; this can usually be initiated by the patient without any specific medical documentation. PGD screens IVF embryos for chromosomal abnormality prior to returning them to the womb.	Depends on age, number of healthy embryos transferred, and clinic's success rates. Pregnancy success rates for each embryo transferred are about 38% for women under 35, 25% if aged 35-39, and 15% if over 40.	IVF only: $5,000-$15,000 (or more, if fees are fully or partially refunded for failure); PGD adds $2,000-$3,000 to the cost of IVF

immunological disorders

Michelle's story

When I was 37 years old I got pregnant twice, but both ended in miscarriage: one at seven weeks, and one at 12 weeks after fetal heartbeat was established.

My doctor said, "Just keep trying, you'll eventually succeed." Of course, that's the worst advice for someone with an immunological problem, which often only gets worse. She didn't test for anything, and at that point I wasn't knowledgeable, so didn't ask.

I went to a top fertility specialist who did the whole workup. All he found was that I had a thin endometrium. But he couldn't explain why. I wanted a scientific reason why my endometrium might be thin, or why it would cause miscarriage. He told me the only treatment for a thin endometrium was estrogen. For months I went through cycles of treatment, then testing, then higher-dose treatment, then testing... But it had no effect. So he sat me down and said, "You will never be able to carry a baby." He told us our only option was surrogacy.

That news really crushed me. I grieved that I would never be able to have my own baby, carry it through pregnancy, and then breastfeed it. But at the same time I maintained a glimmer of hope from the fact that he hadn't been able to explain what caused my problem. There was no science behind it, which left me unconvinced that it was the last word. I hoped there was a chance that if someone could find the reason, maybe they could also find the cure.

I started researching thin lining, and ultimately found a great reproductive immunologist. His name came up on a lot of websites and electronic bulletin boards, and he sounded like he did amazing things. I e-mailed him on the Sunday of a three-day weekend, and he e-mailed me back the very next day (which was Labor Day)! He wrote, "Don't do anything until you talk to me. Your symptoms are not uncommon to women I've had success with. I think I can help you."

He diagnosed several immune-related issues, including antibodies that could explain the thin endometrium. He put me on all sorts of things: IVIG, baby aspirin, heparin, immunization with my husband's white blood cells... I did it all.

I got pregnant easily twice, and have two healthy girls. I had early bleeding with both pregnancies, but felt sure it would be okay. My specialist treats all patients like they're high-risk, which I like – I felt like someone was listening to me, and watching everything. I was on e-mail with him a lot, and saw supporting doctors as often as once a week.

My experience convinced me that a specialist is worth the extra cost – they know the things that matter. For example, my specialist wanted tissue from the D&Cs I had with my two miscarriages, which labs apparently keep. I asked my regular doctor, but she said the lab didn't keep them – I don't think she was trying to mislead me, she just didn't know (though she didn't admit she didn't know, so did mislead me). Then I spoke to the lab directly, and they also said they didn't have them. But when my specialist sent the lab a letter, they produced both samples! My specialist got a lot of useful information from those samples.

I don't know if I have two children because it was just my time, or because of all the treatments. But things turned out happily in my case because rather than taking a doctor's prognosis as the last word, I kept looking for answers that made sense to me.

immunological disorders

Immunology is the branch of medicine dealing with the immune system, such as immunity to disease or allergic reaction. Reproductive immunologists specialize in the immune system as it pertains to pregnancy – they focus on immune response that malfunctions, thereby harming a pregnancy. These doctors identify, study, and treat these disorders, with many respected doctors and centers achieving impressive success rates.

In the past, the cause of recurrent miscarriage was found in less than half of all cases investigated. However, recent advances in reproductive immunology are finding that immunological disorders are responsible for many cases of recurrent miscarriage that were previously unexplained. Of recurrent miscarriages for which a cause remains elusive, it is suspected that many could be due to immunological factors which are not yet clear, or for which tests have not yet been developed. Immunologic causes are thought to be responsible for 25-30% of recurrent pregnancy losses.

Self-assessment

Take a moment now to complete the immunological self-assessment questionnaire below. Following the questionnaire is a discussion of immunological disorders associated with pregnancy loss.

Self-assessment: immunological disorders

(Tick the box for Yes)

1. *Do you or your close family* have a history of clotting problems, heart disease, or stroke before the age of 50?* ☐
2. *Are you prone to skin rashes or migraine headaches?* ☐
3. *Have you had previous immune problems (e.g. rheumatoid arthritis, lupus), or any thyroid disorder?* ☐
4. *Do you or your family* have the MTHFR gene mutation?* ☐
5. *Have you experienced infertility?* ☐
6. *Have you had a pregnancy where ultrasound showed slow growth after seven weeks, clots in the placenta, placental insufficiency, or intrauterine growth restriction?* ☐
7. *Have you had two or more miscarriages after eight weeks where genetic causes were ruled out?* ☐
8. *Have you miscarried after proof of heartbeat where genetic causes were ruled out, or had two or more unexplained losses after proof of heartbeat?* ☐
9. *Have you had two unexplained losses after 12 weeks?* ☐
10. *Have you had unexplained second or third trimester loss?* ☐
11. *Do you or anyone in your close family* have a history of three or more unexplained miscarriages?* ☐
12. *Have you ever had pre-eclampsia, placental insufficiency or an unexplained stillbirth?* ☐

---

* Grandparents, parents, siblings, aunts, uncles, or first cousins directly related to you by blood, not marriage (i.e. descended from a common ancestor).

Interpreting the results

If you answered No to each of these questions

There is no reason to think you are at greater risk of an immunologic disorder, and you can skip directly to the next self-assessment chapter, *Anatomical Abnormalities*.

If you answered Yes to any of these questions

Reading the remainder of this chapter will help you better understand whether you might be at increased risk for an immunological disorder.

An in-depth look at immunological disorders

Of all the conditions leading to recurrent miscarriage, immunological disorders are the most complicated (the chapter on anatomical abnormalities will be a complete breeze compared to this one). I have tried to cut through masses of medical research and technical information to present an understandable summary of the current landscape of reproductive immunology.

Immunological disorders associated with pregnancy loss can be broadly divided into two types: autoimmune and alloimmune disorders:

Autoimmune disorders. These malfunctions cause the immune system to turn against itself (as seen in diseases like lupus and type-1 diabetes), attacking the body's own organs and tissues.

Alloimmune disorders. These disorders cause the immune system to attack tissues or cells it identifies as dangerous or foreign. While attacking foreign cells is a normal function of the immune system, the disorder arises when the immune system mistakenly sees the pregnancy as dangerous and attacks it.

The immune system is one of the most intricate and complex systems in the body, and reproductive immunology is a young and dynamic field of medicine. Researchers the world over are looking at all different aspects of these problems in all different ways. This means that the knowledge base in this field is expanding rapidly, with exciting techniques and treatments being developed and improved. However, it also means that results, treatments, and success rates are difficult to compare; those that *are* comparable often come to opposite conclusions.

Reproductive immunology is made even more complicated by the fact that most of the mechanisms that govern maternal-fetal exchange are not fully understood, and some are not understood at all. Although there is general agreement on a few immunological conditions and treatments, most immunological causes of recurrent pregnancy loss (and their treatments) are considered unproven, theoretical, or experimental.

So despite successful results attained by many reproductive immunology centers, there are also many well-respected doctors and researchers who maintain that the results are not as they seem. Opponents range from skeptics, who say it is unclear how (or even if) the treatments work, to outright opponents, who insist treatments actually make things worse and that some reproductive immunologists are acting irresponsibly.

If even the experts disagree on the biological mechanisms that underpin reproductive immunology, a regular person could never hope to come to a clear view on the subject, right?

I don't think that's necessarily true, and my second story (recounted at the beginning of *Learning From Your Miscarriage History*) is an example of how useful it can be to do your own research and determine what resonates with you, and what path you want to pursue.

If you happen to have a history of unexplained recurrent miscarriage, then an immunological disorder could very well be the cause. However, because many health care professionals question the very existence of immunological problems, it can be difficult to get the information, testing, or support you might want. When making up your own mind about the legitimacy of these disorders, it is worth bearing two things in mind: first, that there is indisputable proof that women *do* produce immune responses against their pregnancies, and second, that *how* something works is less important than *how well* it works:

Proof of maternal immune response against pregnancy. Despite it seeming somehow "unnatural," mothers *do* sometimes produce immune responses against their pregnancies, and Rh disease is a perfect example. Human blood types are classified as positive or negative, with about 15% of the population having a negative blood type. Rh disease is caused when an Rh-negative mother's immune system identifies Rh-positive fetal blood cells as "non-self" and destroys them; severe Rh disease (though extremely rare today because of education and medication) can result in fetal death. Before effective treatment was introduced nearly 40 years ago, 20,000 babies were born in the US every year with Rh disease. No one disputes that this is a maternal immune response against pregnancy that can lead to fetal death. Couldn't there be others?

How something works is not as important as how well it works. There is much objection to the experimental nature of immunological treatments. Unfortunately, until immunological disorders are proven and described as "defined conditions," treatment will be termed experimental. This does not mean it is ineffective or dangerous (though it can be both, and careful evaluation and consideration are required before embarking on any experimental protocol). Also, some treatments have been shown to work "no better than a placebo." But the fact is that even a placebo (sugar pill) can have a powerful effect for reasons that are not known (see *The Power of Love*). Most of us probably prefer to focus on the women who walk in and out of specialist clinics: if women have a 20% chance of successful pregnancy when they walk in, and 80% of those women are walking out with a baby, then that is as compelling an argument as most of us would require. Whether the success is due to the treatments themselves, or is an effect of "the power of love" is largely irrelevant.

Autoimmune problems linked to recurrent loss

The immune system is always on, protecting us from infection and disease. It does this by producing antibodies, which are produced by special white blood cells to fight disease and infection by attacking anything identified as "non-self" (germs, bacteria, cancer cells, etc).

However, in cases where the immune system cannot properly differentiate between "self" and "non-self," it can produce a defensive response against "self" (called an autoimmune response); the importance of these disorders in causing recurrent miscarriage has been firmly established.

There are four autoimmune problems associated with recurrent miscarriage: anti-phospholipid syndrome, inherited thrombophilia, antinuclear antibodies, and anti-thyroid antibodies. These are discussed in turn below.

Anti-phospholipid syndrome (APS)

Anti-phospholipid syndrome (APS) is essentially a blood clotting disorder associated with pregnancy loss in all three trimesters. It is the most widely recognized and agreed of all reproductive immunologic disorders, and is thought to be responsible for 15-20% of recurrent miscarriages. APS is associated with both early and late pregnancy loss, and can lead to miscarriage, intrauterine death, stillbirth, or neonatal death.

In the body, cell walls are made up of a mosaic of components, including phospholipids which are key to proper blood clotting, and which are involved in embryo attachment and growth of the placenta. In anti-phospholipid syndrome, the body malfunctions, producing antibodies against these important phospholipids (called "anti-phospholipid antibodies," or APA). It is thought that APA interferes with the placenta's natural ability to prevent blood clots forming on its surface; resultant clots restrict blood flow and deprive the fetus of oxygen and nutrients (observed as fetal wasting, which is essentially starvation). It also hampers the placenta's ability to burrow into maternal tissues, something essential to its survival.

APA can lead to miscarriage or – if the blockage is less severe and the pregnancy continues – to the birth of an underweight or underdeveloped baby. Anti-phospholipid antibodies are associated with miscarriage, placental blood clots, small placentas, pre-eclampsia, premature labor, and undernourished babies.

Without treatment, women with APS have a miscarriage rate as high as 90%. Luckily, treatment is straightforward and effective.

Testing

Although anti-phospholipid antibodies themselves do not cause miscarriage, their presence indicates an abnormal autoimmune process that puts a pregnancy at risk. Anti-phospholipid antibody levels can change from month to month, as well as before and during pregnancy, which complicates diagnosis. Since some women do not test positive until they are pregnant or have suffered a pregnancy loss, repeat testing during early pregnancy is highly recommended when there is a history of unexplained miscarriage. Tests for APS can be divided into those that detect the actual presence of APA in the blood, and those that indicate APA by abnormal results on blood clotting ("coagulation") tests:

Tests detecting APA directly. There are two main tests available to detect the presence of phospholipids linked to recurrent pregnancy loss. These are the anti-cardiolipin antibody (ACA) and the lupus anticoagulant (LA) tests. These two tests detect different antibodies associated with recurrent loss. While ACA tests have become standard in some clinics, LA is found more commonly in women than ACA, and few women have both. Thus, *it is essential that you are tested for both,* as testing for only one means that about half the women with APA will be missed, and incorrectly told they do not have it.

There are additional tests for other phospholipids (including ethanolamine, inositol, phatidic acid, serine, glycerol, and choline), but they tend to add expense while giving little additional useful information. Treatment is the same regardless of which specific phospholipid is responsible.

Whatever testing you do, it is important that your doctor (and the lab analyzing the samples) be very familiar with the specific tests, as different tests have different results ranges, and collection procedures are very precise (for example, to avoid false negatives, samples must be collected without the upper arm band that is usually used, and must be analyzed within an hour).

Testing positive for one or more of these conditions indicates an autoimmune response associated with recurrent pregnancy loss, and treatment should be initiated.

Coagulation tests. "Coagulation" is the process by which blood forms clots. Coagulation tests detect the presence of APA by evaluating the time required for blood clotting. Popular coagulation screening tests are the dilute Russell's viper venom time, the Kaolin clotting time (KCL), the plasma clotting time, and the activated partial thromboplastin time (APTT). While these tests all attempt to determine the same thing, some are better than others. The dilute Russell's viper venom is considered more sensitive and specific than the KCL or the APTT, while the APTT returns a relatively high rate of false positives (if you have a positive APTT you may want to confirm the diagnosis with one of the other tests).

Treatment and success rates

Treatments for autoimmune disorders are currently the same regardless of specific cause. As with any treatment, best results are obtained when treatment is administered by a doctor or centre with a proven track record of success in reproductive immunology. Treatment options for autoimmune disorders include:

Low-dose aspirin (also called "baby aspirin"). Started 5-7 days prior to conception and continued throughout pregnancy, aspirin helps prevent blood clot formation, thereby increasing blood flow to the placenta by reducing the clotting caused by autoimmune disorders. This widely available low-cost treatment does not require a prescription, is taken orally, and is considered to have minimal side-effects. Success rates are about 40-45% for women treated with low-dose aspirin, compared to only 10-20% in untreated women with autoimmune disorders.

Heparin. Heparin is a powerful anti-coagulant which is typically administered via daily injections. Treatment is initiated 5-7 days prior to ovulation and continued throughout pregnancy. Its effect is similar to aspirin, though it operates slightly differently. While it is considered safe for both mother and baby, comprehensive evaluation of long-term health effects remains to be done. Success rates for heparin paired with low-dose aspirin are about 70-75%, compared to 10-20% in untreated women with autoimmune disorders.

Prednisone. Taken orally daily, this corticosteroid can subdue autoimmune disorders and increase the chance of a successful pregnancy. Prednisone does not pass through the placenta easily, and is broken down by enzymes in the placenta, so the developing baby is exposed to only trace amounts. However, it can have potentially serious complications, and is associated with maternal side-effects such as weight gain, mood swings, hair loss or growth, and facial bruising. While some women can achieve good results with this treatment, attendant risks and discomfort should be considered. Success rates, when given with aspirin, are comparable to that for aspirin-heparin therapy (i.e. about 70-75%), compared to 10-20% in untreated women with autoimmune disorders.

Intravenous immunoglobulin (IVIG) therapy. IVIG is a controversial experimental therapy in the treatment of recurrent miscarriage. It is derived from pooled blood from thousands of donors that is washed and processed; the resultant clear blend infuses the mother with a mixture of antibodies. It is thought that IVIG works by temporarily providing a variety of blocking antibodies that protect the pregnancy from rejection and suppress the toxic action of natural killer cells, which will be discussed later in this chapter. This effect lasts about a month, and treatment is most effective if it begins 7-10 days prior to conception and is continued for 3-6 months.

IVIG is given intravenously up to once each month, on one to three consecutive days depending upon the woman's particular needs. The treatment requires two to four hours to administer; faster delivery times are associated with increased side effects such as headache and nausea.

Some studies report IVIG success rates as high as 70-75% for high-risk women who did not respond to other therapies, compared to 10-20% in untreated women with autoimmune disorders.

Because IVIG undergoes a rigorous screening process, it is very expensive. Treatments can cost about $1,500 each, or as much as $10,000 throughout pregnancy. Insurance companies rarely cover IVIG in pregnancy, as they specifically define it as "experimental, investigational, or unproven" therapy. In addition, many doctors are concerned about potential harmful effects the treatment might have on the immune system.

While treatment for APA increases pregnancy success rates to about 70% or more, women with this condition must be on alert (and have regular screenings) for other complications throughout pregnancy, including pre-eclampsia, fetal growth restriction, and preterm birth.

Inherited thrombophilias

"Thrombophilic" and "thrombophilia" simply mean "prone to blood clotting." Anti-phospholipid syndrome is an acquired thrombophilic state, meaning that it is a blood clotting disorder that a woman developed some time after birth. Inherited thrombophilias, on the other hand, are genetic anomalies a woman was born with that make her more prone to clotting. These irregularities are surprisingly common, and their role in miscarriage is still unclear. However, they are thought to be associated with abnormal blood clotting that can harm the developing pregnancy in much the same way as anti-phospholipid syndrome. The main gene abnormalities leading to inherited thrombophilias are:

MTHFR. A common genetic defect, the MTHFR (methylene tetra hydro folate reductase) abnormality may be present in 5-30% of the general population. This mutation triggers blood clot formation and an imbalance in blood chemistry thought to be toxic (poisonous) to placental and embryonic tissues.

Factor V Leiden. This irregularity is found in approximately 10% of Caucasians (but rare in non-Caucasians). It has been discovered in 60% of women with clot formation during pregnancy.

Prothrombin gene mutation. Also called the Factor II mutation, this has been shown to occur in approximately 8% of women who experience fetal loss due to a clotting disorder.

Testing

Blood tests for inherited thrombophilia evaluate activated partial prothrombin time (APTT), hyper-homocysteinemia (HHC; which detects the MTHFR mutation), lupus anticoagulant, antithrombin III antigen, Factor V Leiden, Protein C and Protein S deficiencies, plasminogen activator inhibitor, and prothrombin mutation G20210A.

Treatment and success rates

With the exception that patients with the MTHFR gene mutation are given supplemental folic acid and vitamin B12, treatments for autoimmune disorders are currently the same regardless of specific cause, and are discussed above in "Anti-phospholipid Syndrome – Treatment and Success Rates."

Antinuclear antibodies

Every cell in our bodies contains a nucleus which houses our DNA. "Nuclear" simply refers to this nucleus; antibodies that attack the cell nucleus and its components are called antinuclear antibodies, or ANA.

Antinuclear antibodies are found in people with certain immunological disorders (such as lupus), as well as in some normal individuals (but only about 2% of normal women, compared to about 20% of women with recurrent pregnancy loss). The presence of ANA indicates an underlying autoimmune disorder that could affect the development of the placenta and lead to early pregnancy loss. The mechanism by which ANA causes pregnancy loss is not known, but it is proposed that some women develop an immune response to the developing baby's DNA and produce antibodies against it. The role of ANA – and whether it even causes miscarriage – is currently being debated.

Testing

Antinuclear antibodies can be directed against fetal double-stranded or single-stranded DNA, or building blocks of DNA called polynucleotides and histones. At the very least, testing should evaluate each of these parameters; some specialist clinics run dozens of different tests for antinuclear antibodies on a sample of blood.

Treatment and success rates

Treatments for autoimmune disorders are currently the same regardless of specific cause and are discussed above in "Anti-phospholipid Syndrome – Treatment and Success Rates."

Anti-thyroid antibodies

Women with anti-thyroid antibodies (ATA) are thought to have a risk of miscarriage twice as high as other women. In one study, nearly 70% of women with recurrent first trimester losses had ATA, compared to 17% of regular women. ATA testing is recommended for anyone with a history of unexplained miscarriage.

Testing

Testing for anti-thyroid antibodies is carried out via a blood test which assesses increased levels of anti-thyroglobulin and anti-thyroid peroxidase antibodies. Increased levels of either are linked to increased miscarriage rate. Testing should be done using the most sensitive tests, which are called ELISA (enzyme-linked immunosorbent assay), or gel agglutination tests. If a less sensitive test called the hemagglutination blood test is used, about one out of every five women that has anti-thyroid antibodies will be missed.

Treatment and success rates

Treatments for autoimmune disorders are currently the same regardless of specific cause and are discussed above in "Anti-phospholipid Syndrome – Treatment and Success Rates."

Alloimmune problems linked to recurrent pregnancy loss

A functioning immune system protects the body from infection by rejecting cells or tissue identified as foreign ("non-self"). However, healthy immune systems make an exception when they allow a pregnancy to develop – the placenta and baby are not "self," but a combination of "self" and paternal genes. While the mechanism is not known, the immune system gives the pregnancy a privileged status that allows it to escape rejection. In some women, however, this privileged status is not properly established, and the pregnancy *is* rejected.

While a number of different theories have been proposed as to how a pregnancy achieves privileged status, it is generally thought that blocking antibodies shield a developing pregnancy from immune system response, allowing the placenta to maintain privileged status. Blocking antibodies are also thought to suppress the immune system's natural killer (NK) cells so the pregnancy can survive. Natural killer cells are special white blood cells that attack "non-self" – specifically cancer cells. Some women with recurrent miscarriage have been found to have abnormally high levels of NK cells, leading some researchers to believe that these women produce an immune response that attacks the developing pregnancy as though it were a cancer.

Current theories identify three alloimmune causes of recurrent miscarriage: HLA similarity, elevated levels of natural killer cells, and embryo toxicity. These conditions are detailed below.

HLA similarity

Each cell in the body carries information labels identifying it as "self." These markers are called HLA, for "human leukocyte antigen." There are five pairs of markers, with one marker in each pair received from the father, and the other from the mother.

Placental cells also have these markers, though they are different from the mother's own markers, as half of them are from the baby's father. It is thought that protection of the developing pregnancy is sparked by the mother's immune system identifying the pregnancy as "foreign, but friend." Natural killer cells are supposed to afford the placenta privileged status, and not attack it.

Investigation into how this mechanism malfunctions focuses on whether some placental cells may not have the appropriate marker, or some NK cells may not recognize it.

In this most controversial of theories, it is suggested that in some cases maternal and paternal HLA types may be too similar. It is proposed that one part of the mother's immune system fails to initiate pregnancy protection because the developing baby is not sufficiently different, while another part of her immune attacks it because it is too different.

Testing

Specialists who treat HLA recommend that a leukocyte antibody detection assay be performed when a woman is not pregnant, and prior to initiating any treatment. Leukocytes are white blood cells; it is the paternal white blood cells on the placenta that the mother's immune system should identify as foreign. High levels of leukocyte antibodies are evidence of better protective response, while low levels are associated with pregnancy loss. Only women with low levels of LAD are good candidates for treatment.

Treatment and success rates

The problem of HLA similarity is treated by attempting to increase a woman's immune response to her partner's HLA markers:

Lymphocyte immune therapy. Inoculation with a large amount of paternal blood cells is proposed to set off a woman's protective immune response to his genetic material, and increase her immune system's future sensitivity to his genetic markers. It is hoped this increased sensitivity will cause the pregnancy to be identified as foreign and be given the privileged status it normally enjoys, disengaging natural killer cell response. Immunization is done prior to conception, and generally requires two or more treatments. Success rates of 60-80% are claimed, compared to 50% in untreated women. *Note: The FDA (Food and Drug Administration) has limited the use of this therapy to specific clinical investigations under special license.*

Elevated levels of natural killer cells

As previously discussed, natural killer (NK) cells are the body's defense against cancer cells. In a healthy pregnancy, NK cell activity is significantly reduced so the pregnancy is not attacked. The mechanisms that restrain natural killer cell activity in normal pregnancy are not known. Nor is it known how this process malfunctions in pregnancies that evidence abnormally high levels of NK cells. What is known is that high levels of natural killer cells are associated with higher rates of infertility and miscarriage.

Testing

Levels of natural killer cells can be determined by a simple blood test. NK cells are isolated (removed) from the rest of the blood, and placed in a culture to see how they react to embryonic cells (mouse embryos at the two-cell stage). Although some doctors refute that natural killer cells are responsible for pregnancy loss, studies have shown compelling evidence that they are. In as many as half of women with recurrent miscarriage, the isolated NK cells attack and kill the embryonic cells; NK cells of women with normal pregnancy histories do not show this effect.

Treatment and success rates

For elevated levels of NK cells, treatment with progesterone therapy is relatively safe, simple, and inexpensive, and early results indicate that it is effective; another option is the experimental therapy of IVIG:

Progesterone therapy. Natural killer cells have receptors for the hormone progesterone; when progesterone levels are sufficiently high, the hormone is thought to attach to NK cells and suppress their action. In pregnancy, the body produces increased levels of progesterone; if this is not working well, then high doses of progesterone can be given in the hope that it will confer protection by quieting NK cells. One study has shown twice-daily vaginal progesterone suppositories to be effective.

IVIG. Discussed in "Anti-phospholipid Syndrome – Treatment and Success Rates," above.

There is as yet no information on pregnancy failure rates for women with elevated levels of NK cells, or on success rates after treatment.

Embryo toxicity

Embryo toxicity factor (ETF) is an immunological reaction against the embryo. This results when white blood cells produce too much ETF, sparking an attack on the embryo. Astonishingly, as many as 60% of women with recurrent unexplained first trimester pregnancy loss test positive for ETF that kills embryos; the condition is also commonly found in women with endometriosis-related infertility.

Testing

Similar to the test for NK cells described above, the test for ETF requires a blood sample that has been processed and left to culture (grow and multiply) for several days. This is added to a culture containing mouse embryos at the two-cell stage, and the effects are examined. If the embryos stop developing or die then ETF is present; if they continue to grow normally then it is not.

Treatment and success rates

Treatment of ETF with progesterone therapy is the preferred option because it is relatively safe, simple, inexpensive, and effective; another option is the experimental therapy of IVIG:

Progesterone therapy. Progesterone therapy to counteract ETF typically involves twice-daily vaginal progesterone suppositories of 100-200 mg each, taken from conception until about 16 weeks.

IVIG. Discussed in "Anti-phospholipid Syndrome – Treatment and Success Rates," above.

There is as yet no information on pregnancy failure rates for women with ETF, or on success rates after treatment.

If you want to find out more without testing

To find out more about these areas, and to help clarify your risk profile, you can speak to a reproductive immunologist. These professionals can be found at IVF and miscarriage clinics, research centers, and hospitals.

While it is impossible to determine your precise risk without testing, this specialist can discuss with you your specific situation and concerns, and provide valuable assistance in helping you assess your risk of infertility and miscarriage (because if you *do* have an immunological disorder, it may result in either, or both, problems).

If you are considering testing

As with any treatment – in particular experimental or unproven treatments – best results are obtained when the treatment is administered by a doctor or centre that has established an expertise and track record of success in this field.

You can meet with a reproductive immunologist – whether in person or on-line – without a referral from your doctor. Several specialist reproductive immunology clinics have comprehensive websites detailing the services they provide, success rates, and fees for consultation, testing, and treatment. Many of these clinics can accommodate long-distance service, so you can choose to "attend" a clinic across the country, or even around the world. Initial consultation or treatment will typically be at the clinic, but a local doctor can usually oversee continuing treatments. Subsequent consultations will be mostly by telephone, with required testing samples collected by a doctor in your local area according to the clinic's guidelines and then sent in for evaluation (blood is easily shipped nationally or internationally via express mail services such as Federal Express and DHL; you must specify that the blood is non-infectious and for diagnostic testing only).

Immunological testing must be ordered by a doctor (or by a laboratory, hospital or clinic on behalf of a doctor). While your regular doctor or obstetrician-gynecologist might not be convinced of the merits of reproductive immunology, there are many specialist doctors in this field who are. If you believe you could benefit from immunological assessment – or simply want to speak with someone knowledgeable about immunologic causes of miscarriage – then seeking a specialist in this field is worthwhile.

Summary

While immunological problems are the most complex of all causes of miscarriage, they are also suspected of being the most common. Great advances are being made in this field, and impressive success rates are being achieved.

The following table presents a summary of tests and treatments for immunological disorders associated with miscarriage.

SUMMARY TESTS FOR IMMUNOLOGIC DISORDERS				
Disorder	**Test**	**Requires**	**Results**	**Total cost**
All immunologic disorders	Full immune testing	Blood testing, which must be ordered by a doctor or clinic.	Identifies immunologic disorders	\$800 - \$1,400
Autoimmune disorder	Autoimmune testing only		Identifies autoimmune disorders	\$350-\$700
Alloimmune disorder	Alloimmune testing only		Identifies alloimmune disorders	\$350-\$600
APS, IT, ANA, ATA, HLA, NK, ETF	Single tests for specific conditions		Determines existence of specific condition	\$40-\$280 per condition tested

SUMMARY TREATMENTS FOR IMMUNOLOGIC DISORDERS				
Disorder	**Treatment**	**Requires**	**Pregnancy success rates**	**Total cost**
Any autoimmune or alloimmune malfunction	Low-dose aspirin	Available without prescription	Before treatment: 10-20% After treatment: 40-45%	\$10-\$30
	Heparin	Doctor's prescription	Before treatment: 10-20% After treatment: 70-75%	\$400-\$800
	Prednisone			\$150-\$300
	IVIG			\$5,000-\$10,000
HLA similarity	Lymphocyte immune therapy	Inoculation with paternal white blood cells (use restricted by the FDA)	Before treatment: 50% After treatment: 60% or more	\$300-\$400
NK or ETF	Progesterone	Doctor's prescription	Before treatment: unknown After treatment: unknown	\$100-\$400

anatomical abnormalities

Debbie's story

I was 28 years old and on my honeymoon. We were young and in love – adventurous and invincible. My period was late, but I had an IUD so it never even occurred to me that I might be pregnant. I assumed I was late because of all the excitement of getting married.

We were not even thinking yet about having children, although we loved them. I was a teacher, and had always imagined a home filled with kids.

But suddenly, there on my honeymoon, I started hemorrhaging and had terrible abdominal pain. I went to the hospital in Mauritius, but it was all a blur in rapid-fire French.

As it happened, we couldn't get a flight home for two days. So in the midst of all the blood and pain, I was trying to be brave because it was my honeymoon. I remember we went to the markets and the smells made me nauseous and sick. I was pregnant, though I didn't know it, and was suffering enormously.

When I got home my doctor took out the IUD, did a few tests, and basically patted me on the head and sent me home. He didn't give me any explanation or follow-up plan.

That night was excruciating. Another doctor saw me the next morning as an emergency case, and saved my life. She knew right away that it was an ectopic pregnancy, and got pregnancy test results as a confirmation. Within an hour I was in surgery.

We hadn't wanted a baby, and I only found out at the last minute that what was threatening to kill me was a pregnancy. So I didn't think it would be an emotional burden, but there's all this baggage that comes along with it. I wasn't sad about losing a treasured pregnancy or anything like that, yet I got this horrible, insidious depression from it. There are so many losses to come to terms with: the loss of a child, the loss of your ovary, the loss of believing you have an invincible body, the loss of your adventurous youth, the loss of your omnipotence. And I think a loss triggers other losses we've suffered. It reopened wounds from the death of my father and the death of my brother. It all took me by surprise, because I didn't expect to feel like that. You suddenly realize you're mortal, which is a terrible insight.

Afterwards I changed completely – I was so fearful. Every month I had phantom symptoms, and was convinced it was another ectopic. I started therapy, which was how I came to realize how the experience had set off the pain of all those losses.

It was two years before I started recovering, and we did not try to become pregnant until five years after the ectopic. At that point I had a dream that I was sitting, filled with joy, under a brilliantly green tree, looking up through the leaves with sunlight filtering through to my face. I thought the dream was about fertility, and that the time was finally right. We conceived our daughter just after that.

I changed gynecologists to go through the pregnancy, of course. You have to have the right doctor who will go through the experience with you, and explain what is happening. Ignorance is dangerous; having knowledge empowers you to move forward and carry on, and rejoice in the birth of your child.

I would have liked a natural birth, but the baby was breech, so I had to have a caesarian-section. But all that mattered was that Victoria was born healthy. Though no doctor ever told me anything about my outlook, I feared my chances of success were really small. I feel so lucky to have my wonderful daughter.

I really believe that if you arm yourself with knowledge you can overcome the past. For me that meant accepting all that I had lost before deciding to go on to try again.

anatomical abnormalities

In order for a fertilized egg to implant, grow, and develop to full term, there must be a nourishing, protective environment in which it can thrive. Defects in the uterus or cervix that compromise nourishment or protection put the pregnancy at risk.

Irregularities in the uterus or cervix are thought to be relatively common, and are suspected to increase the risk of pregnancy loss in some cases. These anatomical abnormalities are estimated to account for 10-15% of recurrent miscarriages – or up to one in every six recurrent losses. Many of these disorders are easily corrected, and success rates for subsequent pregnancies are good. Anatomical disorders linked with miscarriage include:

A misshapen uterus. Uterine irregularities originate before a woman's birth, when she herself is a fetus and her uterus develops, migrates, and fuses into the proper form. If this process does not happen perfectly, the result can be a misshapen uterus that complicates her pregnancies or leads to recurrent loss.

Problems with the uterine lining. Recurrent loss can be the consequence of anything that interferes with blood circulation to the endometrium (the uterine lining nourishing the developing baby). While conditions such as fibroids and polyps are relatively common, they can sometimes pose a problem.

An incompetent cervix. Some women have a cervix unable to hold the developing baby. This problem only affects pregnancies that have progressed beyond 14 or 15 weeks.

Tubal malfunction. Rarely, tubal malfunction or reduced access to the uterus can result in a pregnancy that develops outside the womb (as in Debbie's case with the ectopic pregnancy).

The diagram below of a normal uterus, cervix, endometrium, and fallopian tubes may help you visualize the anatomical disorders discussed in this chapter.

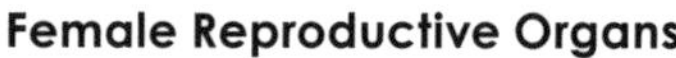
Female Reproductive Organs

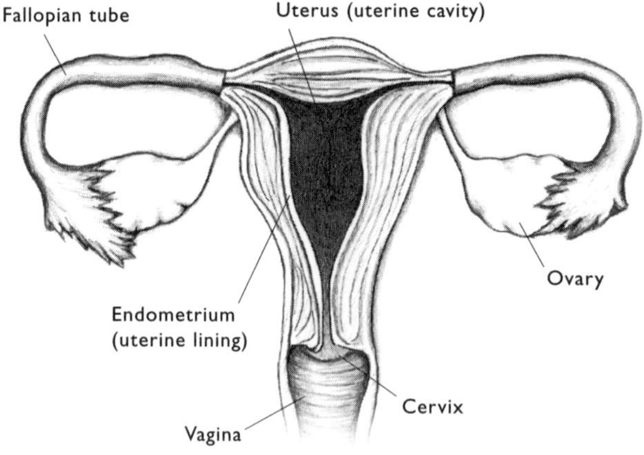

Self-assessment

The following questionnaire should help you determine whether any anatomical conditions might be relevant to you. Following the questionnaire is a more detailed discussion of anatomical abnormalities, along with associated tests and treatments.

Self-assessment: anatomical abnormalities

(Tick the box for Yes)

1. *Did your mother take DES (a "miscarriage medication" prescribed until the early 1970s) when pregnant with you?* ☐
2. *Were you born missing a kidney?* ☐
3. *Have you ever been told you have two cervixes, a misshapen cervix, or a misshapen uterus?* ☐
4. *Have you ever had uterine fibroids?* ☐
5. *Have you ever had endometrial polyps?* ☐
6. *Could you have uterine scar tissue from aggressive D&C or other intrauterine suctioning or surgery, including during removal of the placenta after giving birth?* ☐
7. *Have you had serious uterine infection (such as intrauterine tuberculosis), invasive medical therapy (such as radium insertion to treat gynecologic cancer), or Asherman's Syndrome (uterine scarring)?* ☐
8. *If you have been pregnant before, did you have painless dilation or effacement (thinning) of the cervix, or painless rupture of membranes between 14-37 weeks?* ☐
9. *Have you ever had pelvic inflammatory disease, Chlamydia, or gonorrhea?* ☐
10. *Have you ever had tubal surgery, scarring or blockage, an ectopic pregnancy, or endometriosis?* ☐

Interpreting the results

If you answered No to each of these questions

There is no reason to think you are at greater risk of an anatomical abnormality, and you can skip directly to the next self-assessment chapter, *Hormonal Imbalance*.

If you answered Yes to question 1

Unfortunately, if you were exposed to DES while a fetus yourself, you have a higher chance of having a misshapen uterus or an incompetent cervix. Reading the two sections of this chapter pertaining to those subjects should help you understand how to evaluate and address any risk you might have.

If you answered Yes to questions 2 or 3

You may have an abnormality that could affect your pregnancies, and should read the section "Misshapen Uterus" to better understand how to evaluate and address any risk you might have.

If you answered Yes to any of questions 4-7

You may have circulatory issues that could affect your pregnancies, and should read the section "Compromised Endometrium" to better understand how to evaluate and address any risk you might have.

If you answered Yes to question 8

You may have cervical weakness that could affect your pregnancies, and should read "Incompetent Cervix" to better understand how to evaluate and address any risk you might have.

If you answered Yes to questions 9 or 10

It is possible that you could be at higher risk for a pregnancy that implants outside the uterus, and should read "Tubal Malfunction."

An in-depth look at anatomical abnormalities

For the fertilized egg to implant in the uterus, develop into an embryo, become a fetus, and then grow into a baby requires a constantly increasing source of nourishment and a protective environment. Usually, the uterus and cervix perform this function beautifully. But sometimes there are problems with the anatomy or function of the uterus or cervix that prevent adequate nourishment or protection of the developing pregnancy. These problems can arise from a misshapen uterus, an inadequate blood supply to the uterine environment, an incompetent cervix, or tubal malfunction. Each of these disorders is discussed in detail below.

Misshapen uterus (Müllerian duct abnormalities)

A misshapen uterus exists prior to a woman's birth. From about eight to 20 weeks' gestation, the female fetus forms her uterus, cervix, vagina and fallopian tubes. For this to happen correctly, two tubes called the Müllerian ducts need to come together at their lower portions and fuse into what will ultimately be the uterus, cervix, and upper part of the vagina (the top portions of the Müllerian ducts remain unfused and develop into the fallopian tubes). Once the lower ducts fuse, the central septum (a wall down the centre of the uterus created where the sides of the tubes came together) must be reabsorbed to form a single uterus and cervix.

Errors in this critical embryonic formation process are surprisingly common, and often cause no problem. However, in many cases anatomical abnormalities can impact on a woman's future fertility or reproductive success. Unfortunately, women whose mothers took DES while pregnant with them have higher incidences of these abnormalities.

The main problems associated with Müllerian duct abnormalities are a septate uterus, a unicornuate uterus, a bicornuate uterus, and a didelphic uterus, described below.

Septate uterus

The most common Müllerian duct abnormality, a septate uterus is caused by incomplete reabsorption of the central wall (called the septum), resulting in a divided uterus. The central wall is unlike the rest of the uterine cavity in that it is not supposed to be a permanent part of the uterus, and therefore lacks the network of blood vessels and nourishing layer of blanketing endometrium that the rest of the uterus provides. Thus, if implantation occurs on the septum, rather than on the outer uterine walls, the pregnancy will be unable to survive due to inadequate nourishment.

Experts are currently trying to determine whether a pregnancy implants preferentially on the central wall, preferentially on the uterine walls, or at random. Some argue it is unlikely a pregnancy would implant on the septum when the nourishing endometrium beckons from the uterine walls; others directly refute this, believing the septum initially offers a less hostile environment.

While most experts generally quote pregnancy success rates for women with untreated septates as high as 60-70%, others claim that success rates for women with partial septates are only 25-40%, and that these rates are further reduced to only 10% for women with complete septates.

Testing

Testing for all four Müllerian duct abnormalities is the same, and there are several options to determine whether the uterus is of normal shape. These include:

Three-dimensional (3-D) ultrasound. This can produce detailed images of internal reproductive structures. As with regular ultrasound, a 3-D ultrasound takes a series of images in thin slices. However, with 3-D ultrasound these slices are compiled by computer into 3-dimensional images that are far more detailed than regular ultrasound, enabling thorough examination of internal structures and surfaces. This produces more accurate measurements of volumes and more effective identification of abnormalities.

Sonohysterogram (or SHG). Also called a saline ultrasound, this is an ultrasound performed while saline is injected into the uterus. The procedure is usually performed transvaginally (meaning the ultrasound wand is inserted into the vagina) so the doctor can see the uterus and associated structures more clearly. This procedure is used to look for uterine abnormalities, fibroids, polyps, and scarring.

HSG dye test. The hysterosalpingogram (HSG) test is an x-ray of the uterus, cervix, and fallopian tubes performed after a special dye is injected into the uterus and fallopian tubes. The dye appears white on the x-ray, enabling identification of abnormalities, growths, scar tissues, or blockages in these structures. Some experts maintain that it is no more sensitive than a good ultrasound assessment with or without a sonohysterogram, and that it is associated with increased patient discomfort, and a risk of pelvic infection and radiation exposure.

Hysteroscopy. A hysteroscope is a long, thin instrument with a light and tiny scope at the end which is inserted vaginally in order to inspect and repair the uterus. To perform a hysteroscopy, the cervix must first be dilated, and the hysteroscope is then inserted through the cervix into the uterus.

A special gas or liquid is then pumped into the uterus through the hysteroscope. This expands the uterus, enabling direct viewing of its interior, and providing clear access to areas requiring surgical correction.

This is typically an outpatient procedure (meaning it does not require a stay in the hospital) used to detect and treat uterine deformities, and to assess the uterine lining for fibroids, polyps, and scarring.

Laparoscopy. Similar to hysteroscopy (above), the laparoscope (a long, thin, lighted viewing microscope) is inserted via a small incision made either inside or just below the navel, through which it injects gas into the abdominal cavity, expanding the space and facilitating access to the reproductive structures. Another small incision is made at the pubic hairline, through which small medical instruments can pass in order to manipulate the structures so that the laparoscope can view them from various angles and perform surgical repair.

Laparoscopy is typically an outpatient procedure used to detect and treat conditions such as endometriosis, fibroids, pelvic scar tissue, and tubal blockage.

Treatment and success rates

Treatment is carried out via laparoscopy or hysteroscopy to remove the septum if required. Successful pregnancy outcome after treatment is high, with success rates of subsequent pregnancies cited as up to 75-80%; this compares to success rates generally quoted in the 60-70% range without treatment.

Although treatment of a septate uterus is surgical, many experts maintain that it is safe and straightforward, and that there is essentially no reason not to do it. However, other experts weigh in against surgical intervention, as it has been associated with high rates of post-operative infertility.

Bicornuate uterus

This condition results from partial fusion of the Müllerian ducts, producing a uterus properly fused at the bottom but branching into two separate cavities at the top (described as "heart-shaped"). Although this condition is associated with higher miscarriage rates, pre-term delivery, and breech positioning of the baby, treatment is not generally offered because it is associated with relatively high rates of infertility. About one-third of women who undergo surgery to correct the condition are unable to become pregnant again because of scarring and damage to the uterine lining.

Testing

Testing for all four Müllerian duct abnormalities is the same, and is described above in "Septate Uterus – Testing."

Treatment and success rates

Medical professionals are divided over whether surgical correction of a bicornuate uterus is advantageous. While some doctors report success rates after treatment of up to 70-75% (quoting success rates of only 30-35% without treatment), other experts quote the chance of successful pregnancy with an untreated bicornuate uterus as about 60%, and maintain there is no significant benefit of treatment.

If correction of a bicornuate uterus is carried out, it requires surgical repair to unite the uterus by removing the wall dividing the upper cavities. This is typically preformed via hysteroscopy, described above in "Septate Uterus – Testing."

Didelphic uterus

This condition arises from a complete lack of fusion of the Müllerian ducts, resulting in a wall (septum) separating not only the uterus into two smaller halves, but also the cervix and often the vaginal canal (i.e. there are two of each, all undersized).

Historically it was not thought that a didelphic uterus would be associated with higher rates of loss, as it is a duplication of a regular uterus; recent studies have proved otherwise. Didelphic uterus has been shown to be associated with higher rates of miscarriage and pregnancy complications such as ectopic pregnancy and preterm delivery, with a live birth rate of just under 70%.

Testing

Testing for all four Müllerian duct abnormalities is the same, and is described above in "Septate Uterus – Testing."

Treatment and success rates

Traditionally a didelphic uterus was not treated, as it was not thought to be associated with higher rates of loss. Recent work is focusing on surgical intervention and repair, but this is still experimental.

Unicornuate uterus

Rarest of the four Müllerian duct abnormalities, a unicornuate uterus is characterized by the total absence of one of the Müllerian ducts, thought to be caused by failure of an embryonic duct to migrate correctly, resulting in its complete loss. With this condition there is also only one fallopian tube, and the uterus is made from only one Müllerian duct, rather than two. This condition is linked to a higher incidence of a missing kidney on the side of the missing Müllerian structures, and also to an incompetent cervix (described below). This deformation has the highest rate of pregnancy loss of all the Müllerian duct abnormalities, with a fetal survival rate of about 40%.

Testing

Testing for all four Müllerian duct abnormalities is the same, and is described above in "Septate Uterus – Testing."

Treatment and success rates

Unfortunately, there is not yet any effective treatment to reverse this condition. Women with a unicornuate uterus are generally advised to have a cervical cerclage to counteract the high rate of cervical incompetence (discussed below) associated with this condition.

Compromised endometrium

There are three main conditions that result in a compromised endometrium: uterine fibroids, endometrial polyps, and uterine scarring. All three conditions interfere with implantation, so are primarily associated with infertility. However, they can also interfere with growth, leading to miscarriage, so are included for completeness.

Uterine fibroids

Fibroids in the uterus are thought to be present in at least half of all women; they are found in about 75% of uteri removed by hysterectomy. While it is not yet known what triggers them, fibroids arise when normal cells from the uterine wall mutate and begin unregulated growth, like a cancer. However, fibroids are almost never cancerous. Though they can range in size from a small raisin to a volleyball, typically they are small and do not affect pregnancy.

Usually, a fibroid only becomes a problem if it gets so large that it blocks or compresses a fallopian tube, significantly reduces the uterine area available for implantation and growth, degenerates, or becomes infected.

Testing

Symptoms of fibroids include pain or pressure in the abdomen, pressure on the bladder resulting in more frequent urination, backache, or pain during intercourse. While the regularity of menstrual periods will not be affected, periods are much heavier than usual, and can be painful.

Fibroids can be discovered during a pelvic examination, as the uterus feels larger than normal, with characteristic hard lumps. Far more detail is provided by ultrasound, which can determine fibroids' location and size. If additional detail or treatment is required, then a hysteroscopy (described above in "Septate Uterus – Testing") is the best option.

Treatment and success rates

Treatments are being developed for fibroids, and there are several treatment options, some of which are still experimental:

"Expectant management." If the fibroids are small and are not creating fertility problems, they can be rescanned in six months. If there has been little change in the fibroids during that time (as will be the case for about 80% of women), then the cycle of wait-and-watch can be continued. If, however, the fibroids have grown rapidly, they may need to be removed.

Laser. One treatment being developed involves passing a special needle through the abdomen and directly into a fibroid, and then delivering current (heat) into the fibroid via laser fibers in order to destroy it. (Pain associated with this procedure is apparently limited to the jab of the local anesthetic needle to numb the abdominal skin; there is no associated sensation in the uterus.) As this is still being developed, success rates are unknown.

Hysteroscopy. Described above in "Septate Uterus – Testing." To treat fibroids, hysteroscopy is paired with a hot wire loop to remove ("resection") all but the largest fibroids. Recovery time is short, and this is usually an out-patient procedure. Success rates for pregnancies after treatment are estimated at 70-80%.

Surgery. For women who have one or two large, problematic fibroids, surgical myomectomy is an option, where fibroids are individually removed. There is a small risk of hemorrhage, which in the most severe cases could require emergency hysterectomy. Success rates for pregnancies after treatment are cited as 40-80%.

Endometrial polyps

Like fibroids, endometrial polyps are growths in the uterus that are usually benign (non-cancerous). Unlike fibroids, which are produced by cells of the uterine wall (i.e. from underneath the endometrium), polyps grow over the surface of the endometrium in smooth patches. These patches create implantation problems resulting in infertility. Surgical removal of the polyps has been reported to significantly increase subsequent fertility.

Testing

Testing for endometrial polyps is primarily via hysteroscopy, described above in the section "Septate Uterus – Testing."

Treatment and success rates

Besides being used for testing, hysteroscopy is also considered the best treatment alternative for polyps. Similar to the procedure described above for fibroids, hysteroscopy is paired with a hot wire loop to remove polyps from the surface of the endometrium. Recovery time is short, and this is usually an out-patient procedure. Success rates for pregnancies after treatment are estimated at 70-80%.

Uterine scarring (Asherman's Syndrome)

Scar tissue in the uterus is most commonly caused by damage or infection caused by D&C or similar uterine intervention, especially in cases where a D&C is performed after childbirth to remove the placenta. It can also result from an elective abortion, caesarean section, uterine surgery, or serious pelvic infection.

In the most severe cases, the front and back walls of the uterus are stuck together where the two injured surfaces have healed to one another, and a woman may stop having periods, although she may have pain when the periods should have come.

Testing

Testing for conditions that result in a compromised endometrium are performed via hysteroscopy, described above in the section "Septate Uterus – Testing."

Treatment and success rates

The chance of effective treatment depends on the extent and thickness of scarring. While historically doctors treated severe cases by surgically separating the sides of the uterus, some doctors now prefer to watch and wait, as often the adhesion will correct itself over a period of months as the endometrium regenerates.

Pregnancy success rates of 60-80% have been reported after treatment of mild to moderate Asherman's syndrome; success rates after treatment of severe cases are lower. There is wide variation in treatment procedure, with some doctors recommending special scissors while others prefer an electrical alternative; some temporarily place something in the uterus after correction to hold it apart, while others do not. Opinions also vary on how much estrogen should be given after treatment to promote optimal healing. As with all surgical interventions, working with a doctor who has a record of success in this particular area can be critical to your own success.

Incompetent cervix

Despite the name, no one is passing judgment on a woman's cervix by labeling it "incompetent." In a normal pregnancy the cervix remains firmly closed until labor begins. An incompetent cervix starts to painlessly open during pregnancy without any warning signs, usually around 20 weeks. The membranes of the amniotic sac surrounding the fetus bulge down through the opening until they break, releasing the fetus from the uterus.

An incompetent cervix can be inborn, or the result of multiple D&C (or similar) procedures, DES exposure while you were in your mother's womb, or previous childbirth.

Many doctors think this condition is over diagnosed, and maintain that most women whose loss was blamed on an incompetent cervix will remember feeling physical pain, which essentially rules out an incompetent cervix. These doctors maintain that late pregnancy loss is far more likely to be due to a vaginal infection that spreads to the uterus, or to the immunological disorder APS (anti-phospholipid syndrome), and that women who suffer a late miscarriage should be tested repeatedly for anti-phospholipid antibodies.

If you do have an incompetent cervix, the condition is likely to affect every pregnancy, and generally gets worse with each. However, treatment is simple and success rates are high.

Testing

While regular examination of the cervix can establish whether it is prematurely dilated, this disorder is currently impossible to predict before it becomes apparent sometime after week 14 or 15.

However, an incompetent cervix is implicated in women with unexplained pregnancy loss between 14 and 37 weeks where premature labor has begun or the membranes have ruptured without any associated pain.

Treatment and success rates

Treatment for an incompetent cervix is called a "cerclage," which is simply a few stitches in the cervix to hold it closed. These stitches are removed when the baby reaches term or labor begins.

Many doctors maintain that cerclage does not change the "take home baby rate," though it does decrease the number of premature births. Other doctors cite success rates after cerclage placement as more than 80% for women whose pregnancy loss was due to cervical incompetence. Women with cerclage tend to spend more time in the hospital, and have more infections and other complications; however, this seems to improve when cerclage stitches are inserted higher.

So while many doctors remain unconvinced that cerclage is necessary, many other doctors and patients agree that the potential benefits justify the procedure.

Tubal malfunction

Anything that interferes with a fertilized egg's progression down the fallopian tube can increase the risk of the pregnancy implanting outside the uterus (an ectopic pregnancy). This may be caused by factors that physically reduce tubal access, such as endometriosis that blocks the entrance to the uterus, tubal scar tissue caused by surgery (in the tube, uterus, or pelvis), or pelvic infection or inflammation. Or it can be caused by poor function – the way might be clear but there is reduced tubal mobility. About 95% of ectopic pregnancies occur in the fallopian tube, while the rest occur on the ovary, cervix, cornua of the uterus, or even in the abdominal cavity.

The greatest risk factor for tubal blockage is pelvic inflammatory disease. In particular, gonorrhea and Chlamydia attack the fallopian tubes. As many women have subclinical cases that escape notice, it can be worth being tested for antibodies to these diseases. Women who have antibodies to gonorrhea or Chlamydia are good candidates for additional screening to determine whether they may have tubal damage. However, before this additional screening is done, the cervix must be confirmed clear of any infection that could spread to the uterus.

While intrauterine devices (IUDs) are often thought to increase the risk of ectopic pregnancy, there is no evidence to support this – today's IUDs are not associated with higher rates of pelvic inflammatory disease. It may *appear* that IUD users have higher rates of ectopics simply because IUDs are so effective at preventing normal uterine pregnancy. But because they have no effect outside the uterus, women with IUDs experience ectopics at the same rate as other women. Thus, it *appears* they are having more than their share of ectopics.

While ectopic pregnancy is a relatively rare phenomenon in the general population (occurring about once in every 200 pregnancies), it is found four times as often in women with recurrent miscarriage – about one in every 50 women with recurrent loss experiences an ectopic. This is consistent with tubal blockage or malfunction that interferes with fertility.

Any pregnancy outside the uterus cannot survive, because the uterus is the only part of the body able to provide adequate circulation for placental growth, expand to accommodate the growing baby, and yet remain intact in order to protect it.

Ectopic pregnancy is life-threatening to the mother, as the pregnancy will eventually burst the fallopian tube or interfere with other internal structures, risking hemorrhage (internal bleeding), internal injury, and infection. For this reason, and because treatment options become increasingly invasive as an ectopic progresses, they are treated immediately upon identification.

The symptoms of an ectopic pregnancy are sharp pain in the abdomen, low HCG levels, and ongoing, intermittent red bleeding that almost always begins *after* abdominal pain is experienced.

Testing

If either tubal malfunction or an ectopic are suspected, there are several testing options:

Ultrasound scan. The least invasive option, ultrasound has been shown to be highly effective at determining tubal blockage, and can also be used to investigate a suspected ectopic, confirming whether there is a pregnancy sac within the uterus, and sometimes pinpointing an indistinct mass (the ectopic) outside the uterus. If there is any doubt about the diagnosis, a laparoscopy should be performed.

Laparoscopy. Considered the most reliable option, laparoscopy (described in "Septate Uterus – Testing") can identify problems in the fallopian tubes, and find and treat them, whether the problem is an ectopic or tubal blockage. Dye is passed through the cervix and flows through the tubes, coming out the ends if there is no blockage.

HSG dye test. Described above in "Septate Uterus – Testing," this is more invasive than ultrasound, and less reliable than laparoscopy, but can give good results nonetheless.

Treatment and success rates – tubal blockage

If you have tubal blockage, you can have the tube repaired, leave it as it is, or have it removed:

Repair. Surgery to unblock tubes is becoming more successful as laparoscopic techniques improve. Women with minor or moderate tubal blockage are the best candidates for laparoscopic repair. Success rates for subsequent pregnancy depend upon the extent of initial damage and the skill of the repair. Realistic estimates appear to be in the range of 50-70%.

Leave intact. Women whose tubes are only mildly affected may choose to leave the tube intact.

Removal. For a fallopian tube with severe blockage, evidence is mounting that it should be removed, as it is difficult to repair and appears to have a negative effect on the success of IVF treatment. IVF is often recommended in these cases, as the risk of another ectopic pregnancy is highest (5-20%) for women who have had a tube removed due to an ectopic pregnancy.

Treatment and success rates – ectopic pregnancy

If you have an ectopic pregnancy, it will be treated as a matter of urgency; although ectopics are rare, they are a leading cause of maternal mortality in the first trimester. (Do not panic, however; only about one in every 2,500 ectopics is fatal, and these typically went undiagnosed and untreated). It is crucial to have an ectopic diagnosed as early as possible, not only because it becomes increasingly dangerous over time, but also because non-surgical treatments are only possible if the ectopic is caught early. There are several options for treatment, listed below in order of increasing invasiveness:

"Expectant management." Studies have shown that about 70-75% of ectopics will "resolve" (miscarry) of their own accord before causing any problem, as they are not in an environment designed to support them. If there is no pain, and HCG levels are falling, then the ectopic is failing and is likely to be reabsorbed by the body. It is crucial to work closely with a doctor or specialist, and to check HCG levels every few days until the HCG becomes undetectable.

Injection. If the ectopic is found early and hasn't ruptured, an injection (usually of methotrexate) can destroy cells' ability to divide and multiply, ultimately causing the ectopic to wither away. In one small study nearly 90% of women required no further action after injection. Injection must be done by a doctor skilled in its use, and HCG must be monitored every few days until it becomes undetectable.

Laparoscopy. If surgical removal is required then it should be done by laparoscopy, which not only detects an ectopic, but also treats it (often during the same examination). Laparoscopic surgery (described above in "Septate Uterus – Testing") is far less invasive than traditional surgery, meaning there is less trauma to internal tissues and organs. This equates to shorter hospital stays and dramatically reduced recovery time. More and more doctors and hospitals are developing the expertise required to remove an ectopic pregnancy by laparoscopy.

Traditional surgery. This is not a good option, and should be avoided if possible. The increased physical trauma of traditional surgery results in more pain and longer recovery times.

Having an ectopic pregnancy means you are at higher risk for another, as it is likely there is an access problem between your ovaries and uterus. Your own risk rate depends upon access constraints (whether physical or functional) between your ovaries and uterus, and the intervention that was done to treat the ectopic. As noted above, the highest rates of recurrence (5-20%) are for women who had surgical removal of a fallopian tube due to an ectopic.

If you want to find out more without testing

Gynecologists have thorough training on anatomical abnormalities that impact pregnancy, and usually also have a great deal of firsthand experience to draw upon. Your own doctor may therefore be a good source of information.

While it is impossible to determine your precise risk without testing, your doctor may already have insights into your specific situation that will help clarify the issue.

If you cannot get the answers you need from your own doctor, a reproductive surgeon may be able to provide more specific or specialized information, testing, and treatment.

If you are considering testing

Reproductive surgeons undergo extensive training with tools such as the laparoscope and hysteroscope, and use them repeatedly in their practice. These specialists will probably offer the best chance of correct diagnosis and effective treatment.

If your doctor is unable or unwilling to provide you with the name of a reproductive surgeon, they can be found through other avenues. See the section "Replacing a Doctor" in the chapter *Understand Your Doctor* for tips on how to do so.

Sometimes time may be critical (as in the case of an ectopic pregnancy). However, effective treatment is also critical. In this case, try to get the very best treatment in the most immediate timeframe.

Reproductive surgeons do not require any specific medical paperwork (or the consent of your doctor) to accept you as a patient.

Summary

Most anatomical abnormalities causing recurrent miscarriage are fairly straightforward to identify and treat. The table below presents a summary of the tests and treatments for the anatomical abnormalities associated with recurrent loss.

SUMMARY TESTS FOR ANATOMICAL ABNORMALITIES				
Abnormality	**Test**	**Requires**	**Results**	**Total cost**
Misshapen uterus (all forms) Compromised endometrium (all conditions) Tubal malfunction	3-D ultrasound	Evaluation can be done by a doctor or qualified technician	These tests can identify the problem, but cannot treat it	$150-$300
	Sonohysterogram (SHG)			$500-$1,000
	Hysterosalpingo-gram (HSG)			$200-$600
	Hysteroscopy	A doctor expert in the procedure	These tests can identify and treat the condition	$700-$4,000
	Laparoscopy			$1,500-$6,000
Incompetent cervix	Medical exam	Doctor to assess if cervix is dilating	Can establish malfunction	$75-$150
Ectopic pregnancy	Ultrasound	Doctor or qualified technician	Can detect an ectopic	$80-$300
	Laparoscopy	A doctor expert in the procedure	Can detect and treat an ectopic	$1,500-$6,000

SUMMARY TREATMENTS FOR ANATOMICAL ABNORMALITIES				
Abnormality	**Treatment**	**Requires**	**Pregnancy success rates**	**Total cost**
Misshapen uterus (all treatable forms)	Hysteroscopy	A doctor expert in the procedure to remove abnormal uterine structures	Before treatment: 40-70% After treatment: 70-80%	$1,500-$5,000
Compromised endometrium (all treatable conditions)	Hysteroscopy	A doctor expert in the procedure to restore uterine surface	Before: depends on damage After treatment: 50-80%	$1,500-$5,000
Tubal blockage	Laparoscopy	A doctor expert in the procedure to repair or remove the tube	Before treatment: unknown After: 50-70% if repaired	$1,500-$6,000
Incompetent cervix	Cerclage	Doctor to close the cervix with stitches	Before treatment: unknown After treatment: up to 80%	$600-$1,200
Ectopic pregnancy	Laparoscopy	A doctor expert in the procedure to remove the ectopic	Depends on damage and subsequent treatment	$1,500-$6,000

hormonal imbalance

Popi's Story

I was 37 when we decided to have kids, but I got pregnant really quickly – the very first month. I thought that at my age there was a high chance I'd miscarry, and I was sort of expecting to. But while my pregnancy wasn't an easy one, involving gestational diabetes and delivery by caesarean-section, our daughter was born healthy and happy.

When we started trying for a second child I got pregnant again immediately, but miscarried at six weeks I'd braced for a miscarriage in the first pregnancy, but not this time; the loss was quite a shock. I took it very hard.

I got pregnant a third time – right away again – but miscarried again at six weeks. And then our fourth pregnancy and third loss: pregnant right away, miscarriage at six weeks.

After that third miscarriage I went to a recurrent miscarriage clinic. They did half a dozen tests, but couldn't find a problem. They dismissed age as a factor, and gave me an 85% chance of success.

So we tried again, and I got pregnant again right away. This time I miscarried very early; it was like a heavy period.

My regular doctor wasn't being very proactive, but I did get her to refer me to another specialist. He did some additional tests, which also came back normal.

So we tried again, and I got pregnant right away. But while my blood test was positive, the baby wasn't there. It was an ectopic in my fallopian tube. Keeping the tube would have greatly increased my chance of future ectopic because of blockage and scarring, so they removed it.

By then I was 39, but they still gave me a 75% chance of getting pregnant after the surgery. Although I did everything I could, including a lot of natural therapies, I never got pregnant again. A doctor explained to me later that without a fallopian tube the body can be confused. Hormones will try to compensate, and can throw the cycle out of whack, for example by ovulating too early.

In the end, I think it all comes down to hormones. My gestational diabetes was hormones, my missing tube threw off my hormones, and the problem of "age" is just another way of saying hormones, because it's different hormones at different stages of your life.

After two years (at 41) I went to a reproductive endocrinologist (a hormone specialist). I thought he was fantastic. He said my problem was my age – that the number and quality of my eggs had declined so much that it would be unusual to get pregnant. Everything I told him about my periods and miscarriage history led him to believe it was just the natural decline towards menopause. He said we could do IVF, but that it probably wouldn't increase our chances enough to make it worthwhile.

In fact, our biggest fear when we went to see him was that he'd put us on IVF. I didn't want to do IVF, but I did want to feel that we'd explored all avenues. We'd tried all the natural therapies, so I wanted to make sure we'd exhausted all the medical therapies, just for peace of mind. So when he said IVF wasn't worth it I felt a big sense of relief.

One time I had a young doctor (who clearly wasn't a mother) say, "Just go try again." Doctors don't seem to say, "We're really sorry. We don't know enough about miscarriage, and can't find what's causing yours. All we can suggest is to go and try again." The endocrinologist was the first who didn't offer false hope. He had a "bad" answer by saying "don't bother trying again," but it was good because we finally had closure and could go on with our lives. I think it's too easy to lose perspective; as if having a child is the only way to happiness.

When everyone kept telling me there was nothing wrong, and that I had a really high chance of success, I felt like I had an illness, like something was out of balance that they just hadn't been able to discover. When that doctor told me that there really was nothing wrong, and that my body was doing what would be expected at my age, I felt a sense of relief. I could stop trying and get on with my life.

I think you've got to live with what you get, and not keep chasing something elusive. And I was ready to do that.

hormonal imbalance

Hormones direct a huge array of processes in our bodies, including those that make us feel hungry, tired, or even in love.

The field of study of hormonal function is called endocrinology, and reproductive endocrinologists look specifically at hormones that affect pregnancy.

Essentially all aspects of early pregnancy are regulated by maternal hormones. Among other things, hormones trigger release of the egg into the fallopian tube, changes in cervical mucous that facilitate the safe passage of sperm, and preparation of the womb for implantation.

When these hormonal processes malfunction, the result can be infertility or pregnancy loss. Hormonal problems can result in pregnancy loss up until about 8-10 weeks gestation; after that the placenta takes over the production of hormones required to sustain pregnancy.

Because of their important role in guiding healthy pregnancies, hormones are a tempting target when seeking to explain early pregnancy failure. In the past, hormonal imbalance was thought to play a key role in recurrent miscarriage. However, as more reliable studies have been done, it has become clear that hormonal problems play a smaller role in recurrent loss than previously estimated. Malfunctioning hormones are currently thought to cause about 10% of recurrent miscarriage.

Self-assessment

The hormonal self-assessment questionnaire below should help you determine whether any of these conditions might be relevant to you. Following the questionnaire is a more detailed discussion of these problems, along with associated tests and treatments.

Self-assessment: hormonal imbalance

(Tick the box for Yes)

1. *Are your menstrual cycles often infrequent or absent?* ☐
2. *Are your menstrual cycles frequent but light?* ☐
3. *Are your menstrual cycles typically 25 days or less?* ☐
4. *Are you medically obese?* ☐
5. *Do you have insulin resistance, poorly-controlled diabetes, or high blood glucose or insulin levels?* ☐
6. *Have you been diagnosed with polycystic ovarian syndrome?* ☐
7. *Have you experienced infertility?* ☐
8. *Have you had a pregnancy loss prior to eight weeks where genetic abnormality was ruled out?* ☐
9. *Have you had two or more unexplained losses prior to eight weeks?* ☐
10. *Is your luteal phase (the time between ovulation and the onset of your period) less than 11 days or more than 14?* ☐

Interpreting the results

If you answered No to each of these questions

There is no reason to think you are at greater risk of a hormonal imbalance, and you can skip directly to the next chapter, *Other Conditions Causing Miscarriage*.

If you answered Yes to any of these questions

You may have a hormonal imbalance that could affect your pregnancies, and should read the remainder of this chapter to better understand how to evaluate and address any risk you might have.

An in-depth look at hormonal imbalance

Hormonal problems currently associated with pregnancy loss arise from luteal phase defect, insulin resistance, and obesity. These conditions are discussed below.

Luteal phase defect and low progesterone levels

The menstrual cycle, which lasts about 28 days on average, is divided into two phases: the follicular phase and the luteal phase. The follicular phase is the 14 days from onset of menstruation until ovulation, during which time the follicle containing the egg matures.

Around cycle day 14 ovulation occurs, with the mature follicle breaking open and releasing the egg into the fallopian tube. At that time the broken follicle transforms into a "corpus luteum" (meaning "yellow body"), secreting hormones that sustain pregnancy; the next 14 days (from ovulation until the onset of menstruation) is called the luteal phase.

The corpus luteum releases estrogen, which directs the lining of the womb (the endometrium) to thicken. It also begins producing progesterone to soften the endometrium, enabling implantation and support of the developing pregnancy if conception occurs.

Successful implantation depends upon the fertilized egg arriving in the uterus when the lining is receptive; this receptivity lasts only a few days each month. If the egg arrives before the endometrium is ready, it will be unable to implant; if it arrives too late the womb lining will be disintegrating into a menstrual period.

When the arrival of the fertilized egg is out of phase with the readiness of the womb for implantation, it is characterized as a "luteal phase defect." This can arise from two different sources:

Low progesterone levels. It is thought that in some women the corpus luteum secretes inadequate progesterone, so the endometrium is unprepared for implantation, or to support the pregnancy. This can lead to infertility, or pregnancy loss prior to 8-10 weeks.

Too little time between ovulation and menses. In the typical menstrual cycle there are 14 days between ovulation and onset of menstruation (menses). When time between ovulation and menses is too short (less than 10, or some say 12, days), endometrial preparation can be inadequate – the endometrium can already be beginning to deteriorate and slough off in a menstrual period by the time the fertilized egg arrives. This condition generally appears as infertility, however, rather than pregnancy loss, as implantation simply does not occur.

Although luteal phase defect (LPD) has long been associated with pregnancy loss, there is currently much debate over the role it actually plays. Reliable identification of the condition is difficult, and treatments are ineffective, leading many to believe that LPD is over-diagnosed and perhaps not a significant factor in pregnancy loss.

To complicate matters, with each ovulation a new corpus luteum is produced. Thus, luteal phase defect is likely to be an intermittent, rather than constant, condition.

While low progesterone levels have often been observed in women who miscarry, progesterone declines in response to a critically flawed pregnancy; it is now accepted that low levels of progesterone in early pregnancy are simply the body's response to a pregnancy destined to fail, rather than the cause of these miscarriages.

Testing

Luteal phase defect is diagnosed during the luteal phase by either an endometrial biopsy or progesterone measurements:

Endometrial biopsy. A biopsy (collection and analysis of tissue) is typically done just prior to menstruation in order to collect a sample of the endometrium at the time of implantation. A narrow tube is inserted via the vagina and cervix into the uterus, where a small sample of tissue is collected for analysis. The procedure is similar to a PAP smear, though may produce increased cramping.

The reliability of endometrial biopsy is questionable, as diagnostic inconsistencies are high. In a study where 60 biopsies were read by five different pathologists, one in every three received conflicting diagnoses (i.e. the same specimens were determined normal by some pathologists, but as having luteal phase defect by others). In a study where the same experienced pathologist read 60 specimens at two separate times, his own diagnoses conflicted in one of every 10 cases.

While LPD is diagnosed in more than 30% of endometrial biopsies, this drops to only about 6% of consecutive biopsies (i.e. biopsies taken one month apart). Thus, biopsies in two consecutive cycles should be evaluated before LPD is diagnosed.

Because of the challenges of diagnosing luteal phase defect, you should try to find the most experienced professionals possible to perform your evaluation.

Progesterone measurements. Progesterone measurements offer a less-invasive alternative to endometrial biopsies, as they are performed by a simple blood test. Progesterone is commonly measured on the first day of the luteal phase (ovulation), and in the middle of the luteal phase (7-8 days later).

A shortcoming of progesterone measurement is that it does not provide information on the actual womb lining, but can only be used to infer its condition, with normal progesterone levels indicating normal endometrium, and low levels indicating endometrial deficiency. However, recent studies suggest that most luteal phase defects are not due to low levels of progesterone, but rather to an inadequate response of the endometrium to progesterone. If this is the case, then measuring progesterone gives no insight into the actual state of the endometrium, as a normal progesterone reading could be coupled with an unreceptive endometrium.

Treatment and success rates

Treatment of LPD is controversial due to a lack of studies indicating any treatment benefit. And while treatments cannot save a pregnancy destined to fail, they counteract the body's withdrawal of support to a dying pregnancy, which can make a fatally flawed pregnancy last longer than it should.

Although the benefits of these treatments have not been demonstrated, LPD is typically treated with progesterone or HCG:

Supplemental progesterone. Because progesterone treatment is easy, inexpensive, and considered quite safe, many doctors and clinics prescribe it as a matter of course. While supplementary progesterone has not been shown to reduce miscarriage, it is given in the hope that it may benefit some women. Progesterone treatment can be given as tablets taken orally, as vaginal suppositories, or by injection. It is generally administered from ovulation until about 9-10 weeks gestation, when the placenta has taken over progesterone production.

Human chorionic gonadotropin (HCG). HCG is produced by the developing placenta, and directs the corpus luteum to continue producing progesterone. Although no benefits have been observed in women given supplemental HCG, it is given in order to increase progesterone production. It is injected every few days from ovulation until about 9-10 weeks gestation, when the placenta has taken over the production of progesterone.

Insulin resistance

Glucose, a simple sugar that the body extracts from food, serves as the main source of energy for cells. But cells require insulin in order to absorb glucose and convert it to energy.

The body releases insulin in response to how much glucose is detected in the blood; higher glucose levels trigger higher levels of insulin production in order to process the glucose into energy and stored reserves. In people with insulin resistance, however, cells do not respond properly to insulin; they therefore cannot efficiently convert glucose into energy, and glucose builds up in the bloodstream. As blood glucose levels rise, the body reacts by producing more insulin. Many people with insulin resistance, therefore, have high levels of blood glucose *and* insulin simultaneously.

While insulin resistance increases the chances of developing diabetes and heart disease, it is also linked to recurrent pregnancy loss; miscarriage rates rise as insulin resistance increases. This is thought to be due to high glucose levels supercharging the embryo's natural process of cell death.

Testing

There are many tests to determine insulin resistance. These blood tests include fasting glucose and insulin levels (easiest and most reliable if done in the morning after an overnight fast), fasting glucose-to-insulin ratios (a comparison of the results of the fasting glucose and insulin tests), and glucose tolerance tests (performed over several hours after drinking a special glucose drink).

Treatment and success rates

The most promising treatment for insulin resistance seems to be metformin, a medication that increases the body's response to insulin. In one study, insulin resistant women treated with metformin had a first trimester miscarriage rate of about 19%, while untreated women had miscarriage rates around 60%. In addition, gestational diabetes developed in only 4% of pregnancies with metformin, compared to 26% of those women's previous pregnancies without.

Studies have not shown any negative effects from metformin on babies assessed at birth, three, and six months of life for height, weight, motor and social development. However, no studies have been done on long-term effects.

Obesity

Studies show significantly higher risk of first trimester miscarriage for obese women than for women in the normal weight range. In addition, "severely obese" women have a significantly higher miscarriage rate than "obese" women. Thus, doctors point out that losing even some weight can markedly improve a woman's odds of successful pregnancy.

Although the mechanisms by which obesity increases the risk of miscarriage are not yet fully understood, it has been observed that as obesity increases there is a higher frequency of insulin resistance, higher levels of hormones associated with increased miscarriage rates, and lower levels of some protective hormones. Weight reduction reverses and improves each of these factors.

Testing

Obesity is defined as a BMI (body mass index, calculated as a ratio of height in meters to weight in kilograms) over 30. The higher the BMI rises above that level, the higher the incidence of miscarriage.

To easily determine your BMI, go to this book's website at www.avoidingmiscarriage.com.

Treatment and success rates

Because a healthy diet and moderate-intensity exercise help to regulate the body's use of insulin and also help to decrease obesity, they are currently the most commonly recommended treatments.

Conditions no longer linked to miscarriage

Classically linked to recurrent loss, conditions such as excessive luteinizing hormone, polycystic ovarian syndrome, hypothyroidism, and diabetes are no longer thought to cause miscarriage. However, they are found with greater frequency among women with recurrent loss, so while the conditions themselves do not seem to cause miscarriage, they may be symptoms of conditions that do. Each of these conditions is discussed below.

High levels of luteinizing hormone

The most common hormonal abnormality found in women who recurrently miscarry is an elevation of luteinizing hormone (LH). The role of this hormone is to cause ovulation (release of the egg into the fallopian tube). When LH levels are too high, it is thought that the egg matures too early, and that the quality of the egg, embryo, and perhaps even the uterine lining are compromised.

While older studies linked high LH levels and miscarriage, more recent, well-designed studies show no difference in miscarriage rates between women with high LH and women with normal LH levels.

Because treating LH levels has no impact on improving pregnancy outcome, experts now believe that high LH may simply be a side-effect of an unidentified disorder.

Testing

Luteinizing hormone levels are tested by a simple blood test that is typically done on day two or three of the menstrual cycle, and then again at ovulation (cycle day 14).

Treatment and success rates

As high LH is no longer thought to cause miscarriage, treatment is not generally offered.

In the past, however, treatment focused on suppressing LH. But because luteinizing hormone causes the egg to be released into the fallopian tube, LH suppression must be counteracted by drugs that stimulate ovulation. Thus, a great deal of time, effort, and expense are required to suppress LH yet enable ovulation. Because studies show no treatment benefit, experts do not encourage this intervention.

Polycystic ovarian syndrome

Ovaries contain follicles, which are fluid-filled sacs in which an egg matures. When the egg is ripe, the follicle breaks open, releasing it into the fallopian tube.

In some women, however, numerous follicles cluster together in the ovary, forming cysts. Although the eggs mature, the follicles do not break open to release them, resulting in infrequent (or absent) menstrual periods. While polycystic ovaries are thought to occur in 20-25% of the normal population of women, only about 5% of women show symptoms (such as infrequent or absent menstrual periods, infertility, recurrent miscarriage, high testosterone, facial or body hair); these women are diagnosed as having polycystic ovarian syndrome (PCOS).

Although recent studies have shown that PCOS does not affect miscarriage rates, it is found in a far greater proportion of women who repeatedly miscarry (from 40-60%), indicating a connection of some kind. Research continues into what this connection might be, and recent focus has shifted to the link between PCOS and insulin resistance (discussed above).

Testing

An ultrasound can determine the presence of polycystic ovaries.

Treatment and success rates

While PCOS is associated with infertility (due to infrequent or absent ovulation), it is no longer thought to cause miscarriage. Infertility treatment for this condition is with oral medication to stimulate ovulation; if that fails then ovarian surgery has had success.

Thyroid disease

Several decades ago thyroid malfunction was often blamed for recurrent pregnancy loss. However, recent studies have found no evidence that women with thyroid disease experience recurrent pregnancy loss more frequently than women with normal thyroids. In addition, women with a history of miscarriage do not exhibit thyroid disease with any greater frequency than women who do not. Thus, thyroid malfunction is no longer linked to pregnancy loss.

Anti-thyroid antibodies *are* associated with increased miscarriage risk, but this problem is immunological in nature, rather than hormonal, as anti-thyroid antibodies are the result of the immune system mounting an inappropriate attack, rather than a hormonal malfunction. Effective treatment for anti-thyroid antibodies must address the root of the problem, which is immunological rather than hormonal in nature, and discussed in *Immunological Disorders.*

Diabetes

While studies have shown an increased rate of miscarriage in women with poorly-controlled diabetes, this is not the case for women with well-controlled diabetes. Studies that compare the miscarriage rates of diabetic women to non-diabetic women have found no difference between the two groups. However, it is worth noting that diabetic women who miscarried had higher blood glucose levels in the first trimester than diabetic women who carried to term (see "Insulin Resistance," above).

If you want to find out more without testing

Hormonal imbalance that impacts pregnancy is the specialty area of reproductive endocrinologists. These specialists can be found at infertility and miscarriage clinics, and in many research hospitals.

While it is impossible to determine your precise risk without testing, this specialist can discuss with you your specific situation and concerns, and provide valuable assistance in helping you assess your risk of infertility and miscarriage (because if you *do* have a hormonal imbalance, it may result in either, or both, problems).

If you are considering testing

Reproductive endocrinology is changing rapidly, with conventional assumptions being challenged and disproved at a rapid pace. In this area, as in all specialty areas, it is important to choose a doctor or centre with a reputation for integrity and a record of success.

A specialist center is best equipped to advise you about your own situation. While hormonal problems are hard to assess and treat, these centers report extremely high success rates for subsequent pregnancy, even with women who are not given any treatment (see *The Power of Love*).

Reproductive endocrinologists do not generally require any specific medical paperwork (or the consent of your doctor) to accept you as a patient.

Summary

Hormonal imbalance can be difficult to assess, particularly if the condition is intermittent, or is one for which there is not yet a reliable method of analysis. However, there are a number of tests and treatments available, and these are summarized in the table on the next page.

SUMMARY TESTS FOR HORMONAL IMBALANCE

Imbalance	Test	Requires	Results	Total cost
Luteal Phase Defect (LPD)	Endometrial Biopsy	Doctor to collect sample of endometrium	Can assess LPD (best done in two menstrual cycles)	$100-$300
	Measure blood progesterone	Doctor or clinician to do blood test	Assess progesterone levels	$30-$85
Insulin Resistance	Measure blood glucose, insulin	Doctor or clinician to do blood test	Determines insulin resistance	$45-$85
Obesity	Self test	Calculation of BMI	Establishes whether obese	Free

SUMMARY TREATMENTS FOR HORMONAL IMBALANCE

Imbalance	Treatment	Requires	Pregnancy success rates	Total cost
Luteal Phase Defect	Progesterone	Regular progesterone injections	No benefit demonstrated	$100-$400
	HCG	Regular HCG injections	No benefit demonstrated	$400-$1,000
Insulin Resistance	Metformin	Doctor's prescription	Before treatment: less than 40% After treatment: 75-80%	$150-$350
Obesity	Lifestyle modification	Weight reduction and exercise program	Success rates increase as obesity decreases	Free

other conditions causing miscarriage

Elizabeth's story

We started trying to get pregnant when I was 33. After 18 months without any luck we had all the tests, which came back normal. Both of us had big, stressful jobs that required a lot of travel, and that didn't help matters. The doctor suggested we do IVF, but I didn't want to. I just wanted to take six months off and forget about it.

Of course, I got pregnant naturally during that time.

The pregnancy was really hard. Even from the very beginning I was so sick that I threw up all the time, and couldn't go anywhere where there was food, including supermarkets! I was exhausted, my body ached, and by the time I went for my first doctor's appointment at only eight weeks I was already big! The doctor suggested an ultrasound.

I knew something was wrong when the technician left the room to get the doctor. The doctor started some long explanation about "multiple pregnancies" and I blurted out "Are you telling me I'm having twins?" "No," he said, "I'm telling you you're having triplets." There were two identical twins plus a third fraternal twin. Now I knew why my pregnancy had been so hard!

Usually I like to do my homework and read up on things, but everything I read about multiple births was really scary. Having twins isn't twice as hard as having a single baby, it's exponentially harder on your body. Miscarriage rates with twins are higher because your body just isn't designed to provide what multiple pregnancies require. And the outlook for triplets is exponentially worse than that. I refused to read anything, and resolved to take things as they came.

And then, as feared, an ultrasound at the end of the first trimester showed that one of the babies – the non-identical twin – had died. I was crying, but I remember the doctor saying, "You probably don't want to hear it right now, but you now have an excellent chance of having two healthy babies, rather than three who are statistically likely to have problems."

After the miscarriage I was really sad. I couldn't pinpoint what was wrong, but I couldn't stop crying, either. My hormones were so out of whack, and in the space of only a few weeks I'd gone from infertility and the prospect of no children, to expecting one child, then three, and now two. There was so much going on; it was hard to untangle things.

The doctor was right – I had enough trouble having two healthy babies. I ended up with pre-eclampsia and was on bed rest at home for the last two months of pregnancy. The twins were born more than three weeks early, but they were healthy and weighed over six pounds each, which is a really good outcome.

Of course, it's amazing how your world view can change in just a few months of pregnancy. When I'd been pregnant with triplets I had imagined a family of five; a family of four felt like someone was missing. I wanted to have that third child.

Funnily enough, despite our earlier fertility problems, I got pregnant again right away. And I was on the pill! I was using the mini pill, and – apparently – a stomach flu that made me vomit for several days was enough to render it ineffective. So I got my third child, just much more easily – and much sooner – than I'd ever imagined!

other conditions causing miscarriage

There are a few conditions linked to pregnancy loss that have not yet been covered. From my research I estimate that they account for fewer than one in every 100 cases of recurrent miscarriage, but they are topics that many women worry about, so are discussed here.

While most factors causing miscarriage can be neatly grouped into chromosomal problems, inappropriate immune system response, anatomical abnormalities, or hormonal imbalance, there are a few factors that do not fit into those categories. Nor do they have much in common with each other. These conditions are discussed below, and include maternal disease and infection, use of drugs, caffeine, cigarettes, or alcohol, and environmental toxins.

Maternal disease and infection

Illness and infection are common in pregnancy, simply because it lasts nine months and most people don't go that long without at least getting a cold. Although it is perfectly normal to worry when you are ill in pregnancy, the most common result of an infection or disease during pregnancy is a happy, healthy baby who never had any inkling of the illness that worried you.

While some serious illnesses can occasionally cause a miscarriage if a woman gets them for the first time while pregnant, disease is unlikely to cause recurrent miscarriage, and most experts agree that a woman who has had recurrent miscarriage will not benefit from extensive infection investigation. However, common infections should be screened for and treated to avoid spreading them to other areas in subsequent tests or procedures (e.g. tests should be done for vaginal infection before carrying out procedures that could spread any infection to the uterus). Illnesses and their link to miscarriage are detailed further below.

Illness associated with recurrent miscarriage

The following serious chronic conditions may cause recurrent miscarriage under certain circumstances.

HIV

HIV-positive women free of AIDS symptoms demonstrate no increased risk of miscarriage. Women who are HIV-positive and have symptoms of AIDS are at greater risk of miscarriage, primarily because of increased susceptibility to infection.

Poorly controlled diabetes

Women with insulin-dependent diabetes under poor control have a higher miscarriage rate, while women with well-controlled diabetes do not.

Illness associated with sporadic miscarriage

Some illnesses such as bacterial vaginosis, toxoplasmosis, and malaria can harm a pregnancy if you get the disease when pregnant:

Bacterial vaginosis

Bacterial vaginosis may affect as many as one in every six pregnant women. It is caused by an organism naturally present in the vagina in very small amounts. Though it is not known why, the bacteria can sometimes grow out of control, overrunning the protective bacteria in the vagina. The infection usually produces a fishy-smelling white or grey discharge, and may cause itching, or a burning sensation with urination. Women who have multiple sexual partners, an IUD, or who douche are at higher risk. In a large meta-analysis (a compilation of many studies), women with bacterial vaginosis were found to have early miscarriage rates many times higher than women free of the infection; they also had twice the rate of pre-term delivery. Bacterial vaginosis is diagnosed by vaginal examination and lab test, and is easily treated with antibiotics.

Toxoplasmosis

If you have heard of "the cat disease," this is it. A parasitic infection, toxoplasmosis is actually more commonly acquired from eating undercooked meat or contaminated fruits or vegetables, though it can also be acquired from contaminated cat or sheep feces when changing the cat litter box or working in soil without gloves.

As with most infections, toxoplasmosis can only do harm if your initial infection occurs while pregnant. Having your doctor perform a simple blood test to check for toxoplasmosis antibodies prior to becoming pregnant can give you peace of mind, as most adults have already had the disease. If you have not, and you own cats, then having them tested (by a vet, not your doctor!) prior to becoming pregnant can also give you peace of mind, as infection can only be passed from a cat with an active (i.e. initial) infection.

Symptoms are similar to the flu, and include a low-grade fever and swollen glands, especially in the neck. Some women may also experience fatigue, headache, or rash. If you suspect you have toxoplasmosis while pregnant, see your doctor right away. Of those women who *do* contract toxoplasmosis in early pregnancy, about 10-20% of untreated cases will result in miscarriage or severe abnormalities; treatment can reduce this significantly.

Strategies for avoiding toxoplasmosis include eating only meat that is thoroughly cooked, carefully washing or peeling fruits and vegetables to remove all soil, washing your hands after handling cats, kittens, or sheep, wearing gloves whenever working in soil, worming your own cats regularly, and avoiding changing the litter box.

Malaria

Pregnant women have been found to be more likely to contract malaria than non-pregnant women. This increased susceptibility is thought to be due to changes in the immune system.

Malaria is the result of infection by a parasite, and is spread by mosquitoes in malarial regions. While the malaria parasite rarely crosses the placenta to infect the baby, it can happen, and malaria may contribute to miscarriage if contracted in pregnancy.

Avoiding regions where malaria is present is the best way to reduce the risk of contracting the disease. If this is impossible, you should consult your doctor about anti-malaria medications. Experts maintain that the risk to you and your pregnancy from anti-malaria drugs are lower than the risks posed by malaria itself.

Illness associated with problems later in pregnancy

While certain illnesses do not cause miscarriage, they can cause problems later in pregnancy, and are included here for completeness:

Chickenpox

Over 90% of people are immune to Chickenpox by the time they reach adolescence, so the disease is uncommon in pregnant women, with only about one case for every 1,600 confirmed pregnancies.

Chickenpox spreads via an infected person's respiratory droplets (i.e. on a sneeze, cough, or breath) or through personal contact. It is possible that contracting the disease in very early pregnancy (before eight weeks) could cause miscarriage, though this is still unclear. However, in about one of every 50 cases where Chickenpox is contracted in the first 20 weeks of pregnancy, fetal growth retardation or physical abnormalities result. Chickenpox also poses a risk if the infection is active when the baby is delivered.

If you are unsure whether you have ever had Chickenpox, your doctor can check your immunity. A Chickenpox vaccine is widely available, and is best done several months before becoming pregnant.

Rubella (German measles)

A common childhood disease, most women will already have antibodies to rubella. If you do not remember having had it, it is more likely that you had a sub-clinical case (where you do not notice the symptoms, but still develop the antibodies which prevent you from getting it again) than that you are susceptible to it. Even so, it is worth getting tested to determine whether or not you have immunity.

If you are not immune then you should consider having the rubella vaccine, which confers immunity in about 90% of cases; this is best done before becoming pregnant.

While some sources insist rubella can cause sporadic miscarriage if contracted in early pregnancy, other sources are equally sure it does not. However, there is agreement that if rubella is contracted early in pregnancy and passes to the embryo, severe abnormalities can result. If rubella is contracted later in pregnancy it is unusual for it to cause significant harm.

Rubella is spread on respiratory droplets (on a sneeze, cough or breath) or through personal contact with an infected person.

Listeria

Listeria is found in animals and contaminated soils, and infection usually results from eating contaminated food. The bacteria is killed by heat, so the chance of infection can be reduced by avoiding raw or undercooked seafood, meat, or pate, unwashed produce, and anything that might be made from unpasteurized milk, such as soft cheese.

Symptoms of Listeria include fever, aches, nausea, diarrhea, and abdominal pain. The disease is successfully treated with antibiotics.

While Listeria can lead to problems late in pregnancy (third trimester, labor or delivery), it is not associated with recurrent loss.

Fifth disease

Erythema infectiosum, or fifth disease, is contracted by respiratory droplets (on a sneeze, cough, or breath) or by contaminated blood. Most people have fifth disease in childhood, when it manifests its characteristic "slapped cheek" rash. However, if the disease is contracted for the first time in pregnancy, a woman usually shows no symptoms, with exposure being suspected only through ultrasounds. Transmission rates from the mother to the fetus are low, and fifth disease is not associated with miscarriage, though it is associated with problems later in pregnancy.

Syphilis

A sexually transmitted disease that is easy to diagnose and treat, testing should be a standard part of your initial pregnancy screening if you have any doubt whether you may have ever been exposed (syphilis can lie dormant for years before entering its final phase, which can be fatal if left untreated). As with most infections, damage to the fetus is greatest if the pregnancy occurs during the initial infection. Experts are divided over whether early infection causes miscarriage, but agree it can cause late loss and severe abnormalities.

Cytomegalovirus (CMV)

Transmitted by infected blood, saliva, urine or sexual contact, CMV has a long incubation period lasting from four weeks to two months.

Some women will have symptoms similar to mononucleosis (fever, fatigue, cough, nausea, headache), though most will remain largely free of symptoms. Once infected, CMV persists for life, similar to the related virus herpes simplex. There are currently no treatments for CMV, though medication and a vaccine are being evaluated.

About two-thirds of women test positive for CMV prior to conception. Of those women who contract CMV during pregnancy, about one in every four cases will spread to the fetus. While it is thought that infection with CMV does not result in miscarriage, it can result in severe problems later in pregnancy, or shortly after birth.

Other illnesses

Herpes simplex

There are two types of herpes. Type 1 (also referred to as "oral herpes," or "cold sores") is usually contracted in childhood, and appears as lesions (sores) around the mouth. Type 2 ("genital herpes") is usually acquired through sexual activity, and appears as lesions around the genitalia. Herpes is an infection that persists for life, even if it is asymptomatic (shows no symptoms).

Like other diseases, risk to the fetus is greatest if the mother contracts the disease for the first time in pregnancy, and some studies suggest that initial infection with Type 2 herpes during pregnancy could lead to sporadic miscarriage, though this is still being debated.

If you have had herpes for some time, the transmission rate to the fetus or newborn is thought to be extremely low (0-3%). However, it is important to discuss your situation with your doctor in order to avoid the disease being passed to the newborn (e.g. during the birthing process or breastfeeding), as transmission can result in problems severe enough to cause infant death.

Mycoplasma, Ureaplasma, and Chlamydia

These common vaginal infections are found in up to 70% of pregnant women. While they appear with greater frequency in women with recurrent loss, a link to miscarriage has not been proven, and treatment is not associated with an improvement in subsequent pregnancy outcome. While it is not thought to cause miscarriage, Chlamydia can attack the fallopian tubes, resulting in fertility problems, so should be treated promptly with antibiotics.

Common illnesses

These include colds, upper respiratory tract infections, yeast infections, and most bacterial and viral infections not yet mentioned. While these are common during pregnancy, and may cause concern to the mother, they are not associated with pregnancy loss.

Fever

Fever in pregnancy should be treated immediately and kept as low as possible. While fever has not been linked to pregnancy loss, there is some evidence that a fever that stays above 102°F (39°C) for more than 24 hours increases the risk of birth defects.

Testing and treatment

Immunity (or presence of a disease) can be tested by your doctor. Ideally this should be done prior to pregnancy, so that you know what you do or don't need to worry about (i.e. if you are already immune to rubella and Chickenpox, you can feel more relaxed around your toddler's playgroup). However, if you become concerned during pregnancy that you may have contracted an illness, you can be tested (and treated) at that time.

Most of these tests are fairly inexpensive ($30-$60), although toxoplasmosis, CMV, and HIV may cost more ($70-$125). Doing several tests at one time can reduce the cost significantly.

If you are immune to an illness (as most women are to rubella, Chickenpox, and fifth disease), there is no need for treatment, as an established immunity means you cannot contract that disease again.

If you do not have immunity, then immunization is available for certain diseases (e.g. for Chickenpox you can be immunized up to 10 days after exposure, even when pregnant). Ideally, immunizations should be completed several months before you become pregnant.

Otherwise, take extra care to avoid exposure to high-risk illnesses to which you are not immune. For example, if you are not immune to toxoplasmosis, avoid all undercooked meat – including sushi – and ask that your partner clean the cat's (or sheep's) litter box while you are pregnant (and forever thereafter, if you can manage it, though it has nothing to do with health reasons).

If you have a chronic disease such as diabetes, malaria, or HIV, then it is key to avoid flare-ups by doing all you can to keep the condition under control. You can still have a healthy pregnancy, it just requires more vigilance.

Drug use

Medications. The FDA (Food and Drug Administration) has developed a rating system of every medication's impact on pregnancy. These ratings are "A" (proven safe), "B" (thought safe), "C" (unclear), "D" (known fetal risk, but certain benefits), and "X" (proven fetal risk). Every drug legally sold in the United States has a pregnancy safety rating which should be reviewed and discussed with your doctor prior to use in pregnancy.

Illicit drugs. The FDA has not developed a safety rating system for illicit drugs. However, there have been studies on these substances, and the news is not good. Research indicates that marijuana and its derivatives (e.g. hashish) cause miscarriage and retardation of fetal development. Drugs of addiction such as cocaine and heroin are even worse, and can cause miscarriage, problems in later pregnancy, abnormal fetal development, and permanent fetal brain damage. Common sense indicates that any substance with the power to alter the mind of a 150-pound adult would wreak havoc on a tiny fetus undergoing rapid cell division and developing internal organs, anatomical structures, and brain function.

Pregnant women are advised to discuss all medications with their doctor, and confirm the FDA rating for any medication taken in pregnancy.

Women are also advised to completely forgo any illicit drugs in pregnancy, no matter how "soft" they may seem. If you cannot kick the habit quickly and completely yourself, there are many, many options offering support

Caffeine, cigarettes, and alcohol

How much is too much? That is the question researchers have been trying to answer about all three of these agents whose negative effects on pregnancy are well-established.

Caffeine. Consumption of more than six cups of coffee per day has been clearly shown to significantly increase the rate of miscarriage; it is not clear how much less than that is "safe." While studies are not always in agreement, some have indicated that even one or two cups of coffee per day significantly lower fertility. Of course, the culprit is not coffee itself, but caffeine, which is found not only in coffee, but also in most types of non-herbal tea, "energy drinks" such as Red Bull, many colas, and chocolate. However, you would have to eat five bars of chocolate to get as much caffeine as a cup of percolated coffee. Coffee delivers about 70 mg caffeine per cup if instant, and about 90 mg caffeine per cup if percolated, while a cup of tea contains about 30 mg caffeine. Energy drinks (which are different than sports drinks) contain as much as 80 mg caffeine per can, while a can of Coca Cola has about 35 mg of caffeine per can. Chocolate has only about 20 mg caffeine per bar.

Cigarettes. Smoking is associated with increased miscarriage of chromosomally normal embryos, indicating a direct negative effect on pregnancy. The more a woman smokes, the higher her risk of complication. In addition, smoking has been linked to chromosomal damage to the DNA carried in male sperm (i.e. the genetic material that will make up half of your baby's chromosomes). So both you and your partner should give up smoking prior to conception to increase your odds of a successful pregnancy and healthy baby.

Alcohol. Having five or more standard drinks per week is associated with higher miscarriage rates (a standard drink is one glass of wine, one beer, or one shot of hard liquor).

Of course, doctors agree that the best approach is to have little or no caffeine, cigarettes or alcohol while pregnant (and ideally no cigarettes for you or your partner for a few weeks before trying to become pregnant). If you cannot kick the habit(s) quickly and completely yourself, there are many, many options offering support.

Environmental toxins

Exposure to radiation, heavy metals like lead and mercury, or industrial chemicals and solvents can result in pregnancy complications and miscarriage. However, this does not mean that using nail polish remover, coloring your hair, or having dental x-rays puts you at higher risk of miscarriage. For environmental factors to cause pregnancy loss the substance must be highly toxic and the exposure intense, a combination that is not typically found in or around the average home, or during routine activities. In addition, many women who are exposed to these hazardous toxins will nonetheless deliver healthy babies at term.

While urban myths thrive, accusing microwaves, radios, computer monitors, electromagnetic fields, and even tap water of causing miscarriage or birth defects, experts maintain there is no factual basis to any of these claims.

If a problem is identified, then its removal is the immediate next step. If prompt or complete removal is not possible, then your permanent avoidance of the toxic area achieves the same effect.

Summary

Although many women worry that an infection or environmental toxin will result in pregnancy loss, this is only the case in very rare circumstances. In addition, many of these hazards are within a woman's control (e.g. alcohol and cigarette use). It is up to you to evaluate your own habits and environment, and to take whatever steps necessary to increase your chance of a healthy pregnancy.

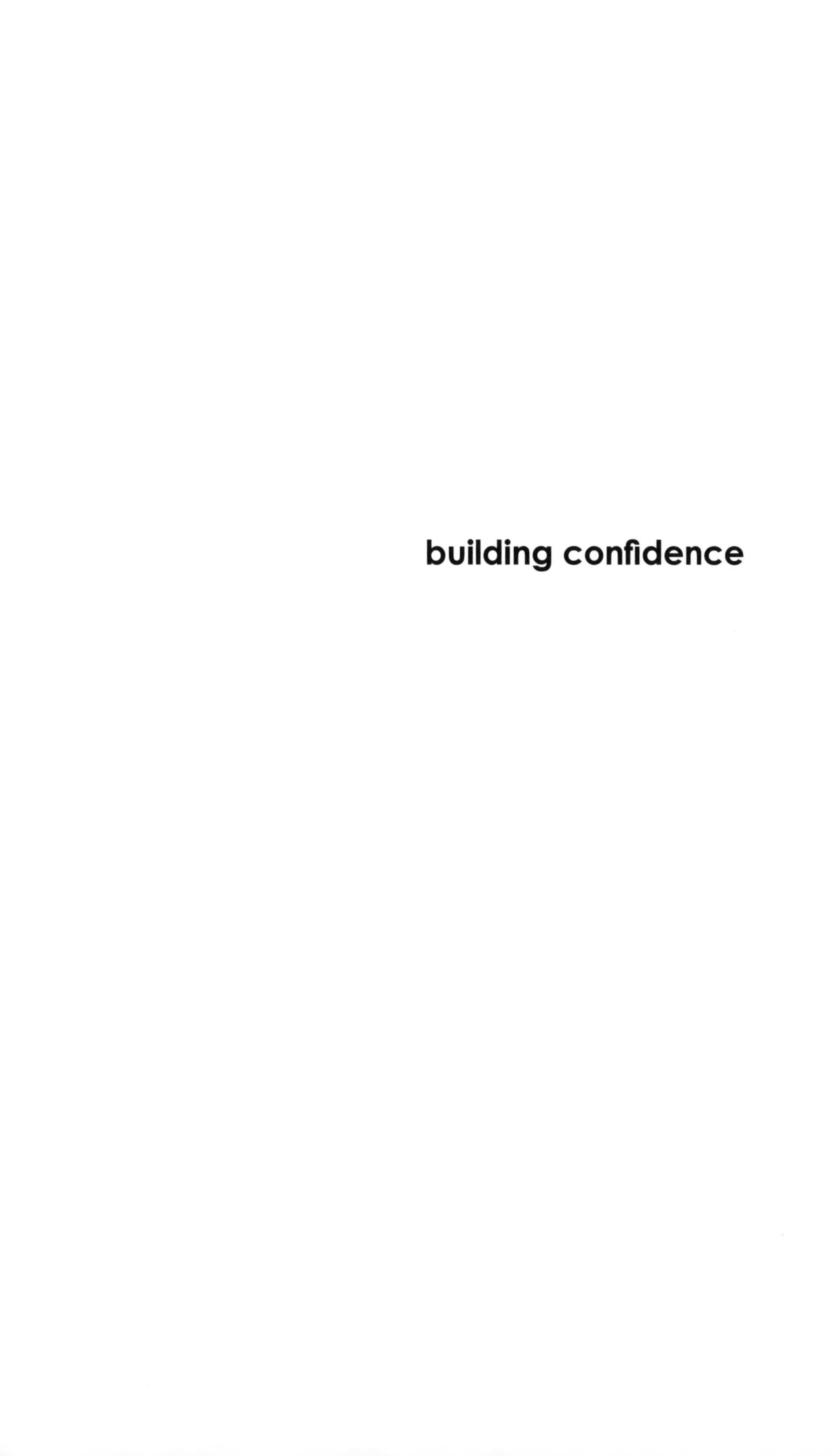

building confidence

the power of love

Sara's story

I was 31 when I got pregnant for the first time. The pregnancy was an accident, so when I miscarried I thought I'd caused it by not wanting it. Of course, by the time I miscarried I was excited to be a mother, and did want that baby very much. Of my eight miscarriages, that first one was the most emotionally wrenching.

I found a clinic that specialized in "multiple miscarriers." They did lots of testing and said, "The good news is: there's nothing wrong with you. The bad news is: there's nothing wrong with you." Because of course you can't do anything about a problem that isn't there.

But they were great. They gave me weekly ultrasound scans, and lots of encouragement. My losses were between nine and 14 weeks, and when I'd lose a baby they'd say, "There's no good reason you can't be successful the next time, though it's hard to see that now."

I never had genetic testing of the failed pregnancies. I wasn't pushy with any of that stuff. I could barely think clearly.

After three miscarriages I had my son Sam. I bled twice during the pregnancy – once quite late, at 16 weeks. But they gave me a scan, found a heartbeat, and sent me home. He was born several months later, nearly six weeks premature. When I went into labor my husband was on a flight home. He got a message from the pilot to call me urgently, and although I had to do nine or ten hours of labor on my own, he did manage to get there for the birth. The baby was so small – I have no idea why it was so hard to get him out!

After that I had three more losses and then my daughter Charlie. She was breech the whole time, so I had to have a caesarian-section. I had two more miscarriages after her. I don't know how Sam and Charlie succeeded when all the other pregnancies failed; certainly neither was an easy pregnancy.

Of course I've looked for any clues or trends in the two pregnancies that succeeded and the eight that didn't. But there's absolutely nothing that I can see.

My grandmother had only one child and several miscarriages, and my sister also had trouble, although my mother had four trouble-free pregnancies. I do wonder if there could be some inherited condition behind our losses.

Now that I have two kids it's possible to put that time in better perspective. But when you're in the thick of it, not knowing if you'll ever have a child, it's the worst thing imaginable. I still carry those emotions with me now, even with two beautiful, wonderful children. My kids are divine – looking at them now, you wouldn't know how hard it was to have them!

I would encourage women to find a support group to help them not feel so alienated. After so many losses, people would avoid me because they didn't know how to treat me. It's not that they were being mean, it's just that they didn't know what to say. It would have been really helpful for me to have had people besides my wonderful husband and doctors giving me encouragement and support.

the power of love

It may seem surprising that love and care play a significant beneficial role in preventing miscarriage, but that has been shown to be the case for women with unexplained recurrent miscarriage.

This is perhaps most surprising because "love," "support," and "care" are unscientific notions, so it is hard to imagine that a study could measure their effects. And yet there is credible scientific evidence linking these factors to improved pregnancy outcome.

The first study was published by a husband and wife team of specialist doctors in Norway. They investigated women who had each had at least three consecutive miscarriages, carrying out thorough medical examinations in order to identify the source of the losses. In more than half of the cases they identified possible causes. But for 85 couples nothing unusual was found, and no cause could be identified. Of those couples, 61 became pregnant again, with 24 women monitoring their pregnancy in the usual way, while the other 37 got increased support and care. The first group went to their regular doctors and clinics for regularly scheduled appointments, and had successful pregnancies in only 33% of cases. The second group received increased medical and psychological support, including regular visits with the doctors, weekly medical exams, and psychological counseling. In addition, they were advised to avoid taxing work and travel, and to have two weeks of bed rest at the time when they had lost their most recent pregnancy. These women had an amazing 86% rate of successful pregnancy!

A second study on the same subject was published by researchers in New Zealand. Group sizes were small, with only nine women in the group receiving normal medical care (these women were "reassured and returned to the care of their family practitioner"), and 42 in the group receiving additional medical and emotional support. But as before, the differences in outcome between the two groups contrasted starkly, with the results coming out exactly the same as the first study: a 33% success rate for the group who managed their pregnancies in the normal way, and an 86% success rate for the group that got increased medical and emotional support.

Why does this increased care and support, which I call "the power of love," work? That is not yet known. Perhaps it has a beneficial effect on hormones. Or maybe it bolsters appropriate immune response. Whatever the reason, it does work.

Of course, these results were for women with unexplained recurrent miscarriage, and "unexplained" is not the same as "uninvestigated." Recurrent miscarriage is "unexplained" only if detailed investigation has failed to identify a cause. But if extra support and care can so convincingly help women with unexplained miscarriage, it seems likely that it could be of some benefit for every pregnant woman. This part of the book will look at ways of bringing more support – both medical and emotional – into your life.

Evaluating your support group

In an ideal world, we would have a perfect support team in place, made up of our partner, our doctor, our most cherished family and friends, and perhaps additional people like a minister or trusted health professional. In the event a complication occurred in pregnancy, our support team would help us through, always knowing exactly the right things to say and do, and always understanding what we were going through. Each member of our support team would shoulder part of the weight on us, lightening our load.

Unfortunately, this is not always the reality.

Women who miscarry may find themselves in the situation where it seems that too many people know about it, or too few, or perhaps just the wrong people. Or it's the right people, but they seem to have the wrong script. The doctor who shrugs, "Don't overreact," the beloved aunt who scolds, "It's your own fault for waiting so late," the friend who shouts across a party, "Look at you – you don't even look pregnant!" because he doesn't know you no longer are. Each comment offered so carelessly, yet hitting so hard.

It is important to take a good look at your support group *before* a pregnancy to clarify in your own mind the contribution that each person can make, and the role they should therefore play. The next questionnaire is designed to get you thinking more specifically about the support you get from the people important to you.

Self-assessment: support from others

(Tick the box for Yes)

1. *My partner and I are a good team when it comes to my healthcare – I feel like I can count on him* ☐
2. *If I decided to have a medical investigation my doctor would respect that decision and support me* ☐
3. *There are one or two people (aside from my partner or doctor) that I can confide in regularly, and rely on to always make me feel more positive* ☐
4. *I usually get support from people important to me, even if they do not see things my way at first* ☐
5. *People important to me would support my decision to seek psychological counseling* ☐
6. *I do not need to "put on a brave face" or pretend with my doctor, partner, or close friends and family* ☐
7. *I know two or three health professionals (such as a nurse or psychologist) who could help me in pregnancy* ☐

Total Yes Answers: ☐

Interpreting the results

Score: 0-3
Either you are lacking a support team or the support team you have is lacking breadth or strength. You are instead bearing all or most of the load yourself, with little reliable support. You need to build a network of people who can support you.

Score: 4-5
While you have good support from some quarters, there is room for improvement in others. Strengthening these areas will increase the resources available to you, enhancing your pregnancy experience.

Score: 6-7
You already have a solid support network in place, and will benefit from the increased emotional, psychological, and medical well-being that it provides.

Creating a strong support group

A support group is a wonderful thing to have in any situation. But given the studies at the beginning of this chapter, it takes on even more importance for pregnancy. It appears that creating a strong support network is one more thing you can do to increase your chance of success.

A support group can be thought of as consisting of three layers: the foundation, the inner circle, and possibly a peripheral group of people and professionals. Your own personality and preferences will dictate how many people you want to involve at each stage of pregnancy.

The foundation. The core of your support group consists of you, your partner, and your doctor. This is the foundation of your support, and the more strength there is in this group, the more directly you will benefit. But "strength" does not come from inner courage or stoicism; instead, it comes from a shared sense of connection and common purpose. In other words, your core group will be stronger if the group dynamic works in unison towards common goals, as it does when you all care about the same things to the same extent. The three chapters following this one explore ways to create the strongest possible connections between you, your partner, and your doctor.

The inner circle. These are emotional, psychological, or medical resources that give you a strong positive feeling about yourself or your pregnancy. Examples include close personal confidantes, psychologists or counselors, clergy, a trusted alternative medicine practitioner, an ultrasound technician with whom you have developed a close connection, etc.

The peripheral group. These are people or resources who can help, but with whom you do not have the same connection, or who cannot provide the same level of support as the inner group. For example, even if you do not have a close relationship with the only ultrasound technician in town, she may be part of your peripheral group because of the important information she can provide. Or perhaps your best friend wants to support you, but has her own issues that prevent her from fully doing so right now, so is more peripheral than she would normally be.

The women who received increased support in the studies at the beginning of this chapter had their regular pregnancy screenings augmented with additional medical and psychological management. Women who have suffered a miscarriage often feel anxious when approaching subsequent pregnancies, and while this is perfectly natural, it makes medical reassurance and good emotional and psychological support even more beneficial.

Your core, inner and peripheral groups will include people drawn from both personal and professional domains on the basis of whether they provide medical or emotional and psychological support, as discussed below.

Medical support

When thinking about medical support, you may want to consider a variety of services, ranging from regular appointments with the doctor who oversees your pregnancy, to consultations with specialist doctors, to visits with an alternative medicine provider. Many experts recommend regular ultrasound scans, as they help women feel much more confident about their pregnancies.

Look for support wherever you can – I was lucky enough to happen upon an ultrasound technician that was incredibly empathetic and generous. She told me that if I was ever worried I could just come in and she would "take five minutes to whack an ultrasound on." I took her up on the offer once, and was hugely relieved to find everything was fine.

Psychological and emotional support

This can come from many quarters, ranging from family and friends to professional counselors, clergymen, and support groups. While each of these resources has its benefits, each has its drawbacks as well, and for many people some combination of counseling and close personal relationships may provide the best emotional and psychological support.

Counselors. Counselors are typically trained and experienced. You don't have to worry about being judged, feel you have to put on a brave face, or be careful about what you say and how you say it. These people provide objective sounding boards, which can be a great benefit, but also a potential drawback if you find you do not "connect" with them.

People who can support your specific emotional needs can have a significant positive impact on your outlook and resilience, especially if you have experienced a great deal of trauma or grief. Women who could particularly benefit from this support are those who have suffered infertility, complications, or loss, since emotional distress is often cumulative, building up over time.

Support groups. People who have had experiences similar to yours can often provide insights that you find particularly relevant. This meeting of "like minds" – whether in person or on the Internet – can be a strongly supportive experience for you and/or your partner. In addition, these groups are a rich source of first-hand experience with various tests, treatments, therapies and approaches, which can help you focus your own thoughts and goals.

Family and friends. Of course, our greatest natural connection is with the people who care most about us: our family and friends. However, while these people can be a rich source of love and support, they are not trained in how to provide emotional care, and can find it impossible to distance themselves sufficiently to provide the objective perspective that is sometimes necessary.

In addition, sometimes our family and friends are so afraid of saying the wrong thing that they say nothing at all. They may think it will only hurt you to discuss such a painful subject. This silence from our loved ones can leave us feeling isolated, or give us the impression that our feelings are somehow wrong or shameful. However, this is usually the opposite of what our loved ones intend. Letting them know that you do want to talk, and guiding them through the etiquette of support, can help strengthen these important relationships.

Putting your support group in place

Creating a support group, or enhancing the one you have, requires three steps:

Strengthen the foundation. Good relationships among yourself, your partner, and your doctor are crucial to a strong foundation. This is such an important aspect that the next three chapters are devoted to developing these key connections.

Create the inner circle. Now that you have read through this chapter, done the questionnaire, and thought more specifically about who you can rely on for support, who are the people that should be in this group? Are there holes (e.g. are you lacking emotional, psychological, or medical support)? If so, how can you fill them? (For tips on finding health care professionals, see the section "Replacing a Doctor" in the chapter *Understand Your Doctor.*)

Consider the peripheral group. Who can you draw on in an emergency? How early on in pregnancy do you want to involve the various people in your peripheral group? How will this group expand as the pregnancy progresses? How can your peripheral group be structured so that it offers you the best support?

Summary

A strong support group is a great way to enhance your experience of pregnancy. And when its potential benefits are taken into account, it becomes even more vital.

Happily, this way of enhancing your experience and improving your chance of successful pregnancy is within your control. From enlisting close confidantes to seeking psychological counseling or consultation with a specialist, you can decide what best suits your needs, and put it in place.

understand yourself

Michele's story

In my mid-30s a PAP smear identified pre-cancerous cells on my cervix. I had a routine operation to remove them, but had a severe hemorrhage as a result, losing something like half of my blood. Back for a follow-up exam six weeks later, they found the cells were still there; they didn't know how to fix the problem. Over the next several years I went to a specialist for another two operations, one of which resulted in another life-threatening hemorrhage, though doctors never understood why.

Shortly after my last operation, we found out I was pregnant. It had been so easy, despite my age (40) and gynecological history. I was happy about the timing, because my mother had just been diagnosed with cancer and given only three months to live. I felt lucky that she was there to share the pregnancy.

We went for a scan at seven weeks and everything was fine. But a scan a week later showed the heartbeat had stopped. So I lost a potential child at the very same time that I was facing the loss of my mother. It was a very difficult and emotional time.

My doctor tried to do a D&C, but failed due to cervical scarring. Five weeks later I miscarried naturally. Because of the operations on my cervix and associated complications, my doctor was of the opinion that I could become pregnant again, but that I would never carry a child to term without cerclage (a cervical stitch), and that I would have to spend the last trimester of pregnancy on bed rest.

Two months later I found out I was pregnant again. I knew I was pregnant right away this time, because I was so much more in tune with how it felt. My mother had started a new drug, and seemed better. It seemed like there was new hope.

However, Mum died when I was 16 weeks along, which was when I needed the cerclage. But because of my previous hemorrhages, the doctors ultimately decided not to do one – they thought it was too risky.

But I was confident this pregnancy was going to work – almost like it was a gift from my mum.

In the end it was very ironic, because I ended up going a week past full term, and had to be induced! Not only that, but they had to suck him out with a vacuum – he was very happy to stay where he was. Doctors said it was a medical mystery. Jack is now 16 months old.

I think women have this innate ability to know what's right, if they can be in tune with that. Trust yourself, have confidence in your intuition, and go with your instincts. I believed in me, instead of someone the doctor wanted me to be. And that gave us our miracle.

understand yourself

If you have had a miscarriage, or have serious concerns about future miscarriage, you may have many conflicting thoughts. Miscarriage, or the fear of it, can create a whole raft of concerns about what might happen in the future, and what – if anything – you can do about it.

These pressures and anxieties may throw you off balance, and you may even wonder if you can make good decisions at such a highly emotional time. If other people question your judgment, you can feel it more sharply than you usually would.

It is useful, therefore, to identify elements pressuring you to act one way or another (for example, if you want to pursue answers but hesitate for fear that loved ones will judge you a hypochondriac). Pressure can be internal: your own needs and fears; or external: primarily your loved ones and your doctor, but also factors such as financial constraints and religious beliefs. Once you have identified the pressures acting on you it is far easier to see the path that is right for you.

A focus on YOU

Before looking at external factors encouraging you to behave in certain ways, it is useful to first look at pressures and anxieties coming from within yourself. Understanding how much anxiety you feel about future pregnancies and clarifying your appetite for action will help you determine what course is best for you.

Anxiety about future pregnancies

Each of us has a unique outlook for future pregnancies based not only on our particular beliefs, concerns, doubts, hopes and fears, but also on our own reproductive history.

You may be confident about future pregnancies, or you may fear you have a problem that could impact them. By examining how you feel, you will be able to determine whether those feelings are putting pressure on you to take action.

Self-assessment: anxiety about pregnancy

(Tick the box for Yes)

1. *I think I will probably have trouble with future pregnancies* ☐
2. *I think my chance of miscarriage is higher than average* ☐
3. *I think I'm running out of time for a healthy pregnancy* ☐
4. *It is important to me to have a baby in the next year or so* ☐
5. *I'm afraid it could take me a long time to get pregnant* ☐
6. *If I have a miscarriage I don't know if I'll be able to cope* ☐

Total Yes Answers: ☐

Interpreting the results

Score: 0-1

You are relaxed about your chance of success, and probably expect to create the family you want without much complication. You do not have issues you feel you must address in order to assure future pregnancies.

Score: 2-3

You may be worried that future pregnancies will be complicated. Reducing your anxiety in specific areas of uncertainty (e.g. by speaking to a specialist in that subject) would probably help you.

Score: 4-6

You have real concerns about future pregnancies, and may feel very determined to ensure the next one works. Anything you can do to reduce your anxiety and increase your chance of successful pregnancy would be a top priority.

Your appetite for action

Some women are comfortable asking for what they want, other women loathe doing so. Some women feel they simply must act to confront an issue of concern, while others prefer to wait to see what comes of it. Clarifying your natural inclination for taking action will help you determine what level is right for you.

Self-assessment: appetite for action

(Tick the box for Yes)

1. *I want to* ***do*** *something about my miscarriage risk* ☐
2. *I can ask for what I want if I think it is really important* ☐
3. *I want to lay solid groundwork for a successful pregnancy* ☐
4. *If I can't get what I want directly, I can usually come up with other ways of getting it* ☐
5. *I would feel better if I were doing something useful to reduce my chance of miscarriage* ☐
6. *If someone tells me 'no,' I can insist if it's important to me* ☐

Total Yes Answers: ☐

Interpreting the results

Score: 0-1

You do not feel a great need to act, and you are not terribly comfortable doing so, either. Taking action is not something that feeds your soul. On the contrary, it may be a source of stress for you. If you ultimately decide that you need to take action, then perhaps you can ask someone you trust to help and support you in this area (for example, by accompanying you to appointments).

Score: 2-3

Either you are not convinced you need to take action, or you are not entirely comfortable doing so. This profile will not keep you from pursuing answers if you want to, but may encourage you to settle for less than you really want. Doing further research in specific areas of concern may help you determine whether or not you need to take action.

Score: 4-6

You are naturally prone to taking action, and are comfortable doing so. You can ask for what you want, and if it is not forthcoming then you are probably ready to insist on it, or to pursue other avenues in order to get it. Your propensity to act will encourage you to do so, and you may crave taking action in order to influence this area of your life. You will probably find that tangible action (such as further investigation or replacing a doctor) is the right course for you.

It's about you

Of course, you are not the only one whose needs are important in this situation. Your doctor, partner, family and friends are all involved right along with you. But while you are not the only person involved, you are the most important. Your next pregnancy will succeed or fail in your body – not your doctor's or even your husband's. While they have legitimate feelings of their own – and you should try to listen to them and understand them – this is not a time to put other people first. In the end you must do what is right for you, even if that opposes what others seem to think you should do. We all know there is nothing worse than looking back with regret.

There is no doubt that miscarriage concern can make hard decisions even harder. So if you haven't already been doing so, then from now on you should give top priority to identifying and meeting your own needs in this area.

External pressures

Your own needs and anxieties are not the only factors influencing you. Input from loved ones and your doctor, as well as pressure from a variety of other sources, can all have an effect on your decisions. Understanding the role each of these aspects plays will help you clarify how best to respond to them.

Loved ones

In the previous chapter we looked at the strength of your support group. If you feel pressured to act in a certain way by people who are important to you, this will weigh on you, particularly if it is not what you yourself want to do.

Look back at the questionnaire on page 175 and go through the questions once again to determine if you feel pressured to respond in a particular way by anyone close to you.

Your doctor

In the uncertainty of miscarriage we usually take our doctors' advice about what to do. But the advice most commonly given – to go home and try again – does not take a woman's unique circumstances or personal preferences into account. While it may be sound advice for some women, for others it may be the worst thing they can do.

For example, if you found it difficult to get pregnant previously, or feel like you are running out of time, you may not be comfortable with the "trial and error" method of getting pregnant again, essentially using your next pregnancy to detect if there is a problem. Or you may simply want additional data on some specific cause of miscarriage and how it might affect you. Or it may just be your personal preference to have more information.

Whatever your reasons, if you want to clarify something about your own health, then that is not only a valid need, it is your right. After all, this aspect of your healthcare concerns the life or death of the next child you conceive. And it is your body, time and money that you must sacrifice in order to get answers. A doctor who responds to a request for more information or testing by saying it is "not worth it" is looking primarily at the monetary cost to you. But it is more appropriately *you* who decide how to balance the costs of time, money, and mental energy against the benefit of greater clarity.

Other constraints

There are a number of other factors that can pressure you to respond (or not respond) in a certain way:

Cost. The cost of full medical testing can be significant. If you have limited resources, you may worry that a lack of funds limits the amount of investigation you can pursue.

Time. Similarly, you might not think you have the time to get the answers you need. Perhaps you are already pregnant, or maybe you think an investigation will not be able to return concrete results before you become pregnant again.

Disruption. You could worry that pursuing answers will cause too much disruption to your life, whether because you have a very demanding job, a house full of children, or simply a strong desire to preserve any sense of normality that remains in your life.

Beliefs. Your beliefs or religion may discourage or forbid the use of doctors and medicine, or suggest that a miscarriage is what God has chosen for you, implying that you should not question it.

Each of these concerns can exert pressure on you to act one way or another. Identifying and considering these pressures enables you to find ways of counteracting them, and opens up the possibility of making necessary compromises while still meeting your needs.

Summary

When facing a future that has any hint of miscarriage risk, it can be difficult to think clearly about our options and preferred responses. By analyzing your own needs and anxieties, as well as pressures from other sources, you can separate the jumble into distinct, manageable strands. Doing this can enable you to assess them, think more clearly about what you really want, and determine how best to respond in order to go down the path that is right for you.

understand your partner

Many women's comments

For women who experience or worry about pregnancy loss, the effect on their relationship is likely to be as unique as the relationship itself. Though many couples will have issues and characteristics in common, there is no "typical" way of working through them. This case is therefore a collection of comments women made about how pregnancy loss affected their relationship.

"I was grieving, and very upset about what was happening. I was ready to give up. But my husband wasn't, and helped me go on."

"My husband thought I was being way too anxious and panicky. He achieved the disconnect, and was logical and rational earlier."

"My husband was fantastic. He felt the loss himself, though I noticed that no one ever asked him if he was okay. No one supported him, and I probably didn't either, because I was so caught up in it."

"The miscarriage changed our lives. It was years before we tried again. Before I had been passionate, but after I was fearful."

"It brought us closer together in some ways, and it connected him more to the kids we already had – made them more precious, and something to be treated more gently and compassionately."

"It was only through therapy that I realized how the loss impacted our marriage."

"We really tried to work on not letting it rule our lives. To be honest, I think it made us stronger as a team. He was very supportive, and driven by whatever I wanted."

"Afterwards, all the romance can go out the window: 'Don't tell me you're going to be away on business while I'm ovulating?!'"

"He felt grief over the losses, but I don't know if it was for my pain and upset, or for the loss itself."

"It brought us closer together because he was marvelous. After a loss I'd be an absolute bitch for two or three days. I wouldn't do any work, take any calls, or even get up – that was my coping mechanism. He would make me cups of tea, look after me, and do whatever needed to be done. He was great."

"My husband seemed to think everything would be all right and that I should just get over it and get on with it. He didn't seem to understand that we'd lost a baby."

"Once we got through the critical time, he became so excited – so thrilled we were really going to have a baby."

"We went through a tough few months. There was so much tension. It was very difficult at times."

"We tried to keep humor in it, and that wasn't always easy. We tried to do things for each other, and to acknowledge that certain things at certain times were very stressful. I got into yoga, and we enjoyed doing that together; it made us a lot closer."

"It took a couple of years to get past the mindset that took over about trying to get pregnant: 'You have to be home on night 11 and on night 13…' For a while there it's like business, and that's grim."

"We discussed what we would do if we couldn't have children, and how that would change our world and relationships. We talked through issues that were very hard to consider and confront."

"The emotional stress really built up – we were demoralized. In many ways it brought us closer, but there's no doubt we went through our depressions, and were too defeated to help each other as much as we'd have liked to."

"My husband doesn't think you should push too much in life, and instead be happy with what you get: the process is more important than the goal. The losses gave us an opportunity to practice that."

understand your partner

Your partner is in a better position than anyone to provide essential support to you in pregnancy. However, he may also be a source of anxiety, much as neither of you want it to be so. This chapter will look at ways to strengthen the support you give each other, and combat the tension that can arise from pregnancy concerns.

Stepping into your partner's shoes

People often assume that miscarriage does not affect men to the same degree as women. This assumption is likely based on the fact that women are physically bound to the pregnancy in a way men are not. But women who miscarry report that the physical aspect is only part of the equation; emotional and psychological well-being suffer more damage and take far longer to heal. This is demonstrated in many ways, such as grieving for the child that might have been, blaming themselves, mistrusting their bodies, or questioning their ability to be good mothers. It is the emotional wounds that make miscarriage so injurious, and this aspect can hit men just as hard as it hits women.

Emotionally, impending parenthood triggers the same range of feelings in men as it does in women, ranging from joy and pride to uncertainty and anxiety. Whether the pregnancy was an accident or the result of years of trying, its very existence will cause a man to wonder how events will unfold, and how this new life will thread its way through the future. Men imagine a future that includes this child, just as women do. For men, just as for women, miscarriage can erase a life that was somehow bigger than any ultrasound could ever show.

And miscarriage gives both women and men a burden that the other cannot bear for them. For a woman, it is having to endure the physical pain and changes that miscarriage brings. For a man, it is being completely powerless to protect his baby from death, and his wife from physical and emotional pain. He can only look on as events unfold, unable to lessen her pain or change the outcome.

See how it feels to reverse the roles: Imagine watching your husband beg God, fate, or the doctor to save something that can't be saved, his hand clutching yours and his eyes full of tears, shock, or fear. Imagine how you would feel knowing that he alone must bear the physical suffering for a dream you both shared. Imagine watching him endure physical or emotional pain so great that he is left sobbing for days, and grieving for months or years.

For a man, a miscarriage is more than the loss of a baby; it is also the awful powerlessness of watching his wife suffer the most distressing experience of her life without being able to shield her. But because a man does not carry a pregnancy, and therefore does not have the same physical connection to it as a woman, he is often overlooked if the pregnancy is lost. Most men are offered only a fraction of the support their wives receive, even though their experience may have been just as harrowing in its own way.

The rest of this chapter looks at what your partner might be feeling, the pressures and habits that might cause him to express things in ways that can be misunderstood, and how to cut through those misunderstandings and strengthen the bond with him.

It's a man thing

A miscarriage can have a huge impact on man, and on the way he sees himself. He might experience a powerful jumble of emotions ranging from guilt to anger. His behavior might sometimes seem nonchalant, erratic, or just plain incomprehensible, which can lead to misunderstanding. It is worth looking more closely at what he might be feeling and why he might act the way he does.

What he might feel

If you have experienced a miscarriage, your partner may be suddenly thrust into a situation where he can feel an overwhelming array of emotions, including:

Powerlessness. If you have ever had to watch someone you love suffer, you may have found yourself wishing you could bear the pain instead of them; enduring it yourself is better than watching helplessly as they struggle to cope. Of course, this awful position is precisely where men land when their partners miscarry.

Remorse. If the pregnancy was unplanned or happened sooner than expected, or even if it simply triggered normal concerns about major life changes, your partner might feel some measure of relief, which itself triggers feelings of guilt and remorse. But closure almost always brings about some feeling of relief, even when the outcome was the opposite of what we wanted; it is a perfectly normal feeling for both men and women, and should not be a source of guilt.

Guilt. Your partner has to watch your suffering in the knowledge that if it weren't for him you wouldn't have been carrying the pregnancy in the first place. Although he is not responsible for the miscarriage, he *is* responsible for the pregnancy, and the leap of logic required to feel a great deal of guilt is only very small.

Sorrow. He may feel sorrow for the baby you have both lost, for the suffering you have been through, and for the way the future has been so dramatically altered.

Anger. Many men feel angry about a loss, whether because of the unfairness of it, the devastation it causes, or the infuriating frustration that comes from having no control over this major part of life.

Confusion. Many people believe that bad things don't "just happen." When something as bad as pregnancy loss *does* happen, a man may find himself feeling as though his partner must be to blame, even though he knows this is not the case. This clash between emotion and logic can lead to a great deal of tension, as he swings erratically between sympathy and blame.

How he might act

While modern men are urged to be in touch with their emotions, people can be woefully unprepared to respond effectively when they are. For example, if a woman was found weeping at her desk a month after she had miscarried, colleagues would probably be supportive and understanding. If a man was found weeping at his desk a month after his wife had miscarried, colleagues might call the paramedics.

After a miscarriage, men often feel an obligation to be strong for their wives, reassure others, and suppress their own needs:

Being strong for you. Men sum it up by saying: "My wife is going through so much right now; I don't want to add to her burden." Men that are relentlessly jolly and reassuring with their bewildered wives can be confused, emotional, or tearful when they're alone.

Reassuring others. Many men find that talking about the loss with others is more draining than healing. To avoid discussions they think could deplete them further, men often assure others they are fine.

Suppressing his own feelings. Some men feel it is not their right to focus on their own feelings when their wife has suffered so much, particularly if they feel angry or resentful. Although they have just as much right (and need) as women to acknowledge and work through what they are feeling, many men will act in a way that leaves their needs unmet.

Problems that can arise

Miscarriage hits men with a double-whammy: it demands that they surrender to the powerlessness of being unable to change the course of events, while at the same time pressuring them to stand solid as a rock in order to spare everyone else worry. This disconnect between what a man might feel (weak) and how he might act (strong) can lead to problems including tension with his wife, lack of a support group, feelings of isolation, and lasting emotional damage:

Tension in the marriage. This can arise from a variety of sources, including different coping styles and being out of sync with each other when going through the different stages of loss. For example, a man may cope by putting on a brave face, and expect that this will comfort his wife. But rather than reducing his wife's concern, a man's resilient demeanor can increase it by making her wonder if he is "on the same page." Women express disconnects of style and rhythm in a variety of ways: "He didn't get it," "He didn't seem to realize it was a baby we lost," or "He got over it much faster than I did." These differences can create tension and leave each partner wondering what is wrong with the other.

No support group. Often a man will downplay his own needs, whether because he wants to spare his wife or because he is not comfortable expressing what he is feeling. His behavior reassures friends and family that he does not need their support, so little is offered. Of course, a man could benefit from care and attention just as much as a woman does. Recovering from miscarriage without any support is a long, difficult, lonely road.

Feeling isolated. After a miscarriage men can feel as though no one understands what they're going through. Whether this is because they are putting on a brave face, or because people assume miscarriage is a woman's event, men can feel as though they are going it alone. Because of this, they might even wonder if their feelings are abnormal in some way. For many men the aftermath of a miscarriage will be the most difficult time they have ever faced; feeling isolated can only make it harder.

Lasting emotional issues. When a man suppresses his own feelings in order to better support his wife or the people around him, his own emotions are put to the side to be dealt with later (or never). Psychologists agree that when grief or trauma are denied or hidden (as when a widow "holds it together" for her children's sake) they require far more time to work through than if they are acknowledged and dealt with when they occur.

Staying on the same team

If I were ever in the awful situation at the beginning of this chapter, with my husband suffering while I looked on, I expect I would be useless. I would probably rub his hand and endlessly repeat that everything would be fine, even though I would have no idea how that might turn out to be true. My assurances would reflect my hope for the future, rather than any insight or plan.

Of course, when a man utters assurances in response to his wife's miscarriage, it can make her crazy. Or not. It depends on the man, the woman, and the timing. Let's look at some of the ways men can react to miscarriage, and how these reactions can be misinterpreted.

"He just keeps saying everything's going to be fine."

What he might be trying to say or do: As mentioned above, this assurance can arise naturally out of the wish to soothe and comfort, or it can be his way of saying that he knows the two of you will somehow get through this together.

How it can be taken badly: Unfortunately, as the baby is obviously not going to be fine, it can seem he is dismissing the loss without a second thought.

How to get to the heart of it: You need to know that he is talking about the two of you getting through this together – that you are still a strong and solid team even on this terribly unstable ground. Get that information in whatever way works for you.

"He just shrugs and gets on with life"

What he might be trying to say or do: Because their bodies have not let them down, men can often be more objective about a miscarriage. He may be ready to move on more quickly than you are, particularly if you take the loss as a personal failing. This quicker recovery (referred to by women as "moving on," "getting back to normal," "going on with life," or being "unconcerned") could simply reflect his optimism that future attempts will be trouble-free.

How it can be taken badly: When we're miserable we don't want our partner to be objective – we'd like him to be a bit miserable, too. If he moves on more quickly, it can leave us feeling isolated and misunderstood at one of the most vulnerable times of our life.

How to get to the heart of it. If you can share some of your concerns and uncertainties with him, and encourage him to share his view with you, you will both better understand where the disconnect arises. Don't take his objectiveness as callousness; he is probably right to think you will go on to happy and successful pregnancies.

"He seems to blame me for the loss"

What he might be trying to say or do: Trying to find a reason for a loss is our way of trying to ensure that it never happens again. Just as women search for a reason and often blame themselves, men can too.

How it can be taken badly: It's painful enough to be self-critical, but it is even worse when loved ones join in the criticism.

How to get to the heart of it. He needs to know that miscarriage is something that usually strikes at random, and that blaming you only makes the situation worse for both of you. Because it is based on a fundamental belief, rather than the situation itself, this issue can be very complex and difficult to overcome; it may be useful for him to speak to a grief counselor.

"He wants to have sex" (or he doesn't)

What he might be trying to say or do: Some men think that making love as soon as is safe after a miscarriage will demonstrate the depth of their love for their wife. Others are reluctant, because sex is linked to pregnancy, and pregnancy is what caused their wife's suffering.

How it can be taken badly: Women can feel exactly the same as men (either they want to or they don't), and when this is out of sync with their partner then things can go wrong. For example, the woman who wants to have sex but whose partner doesn't will have one more bruise to add to her battered self-esteem, while the woman whose husband is ready for sex before she is can feel he is insensitive.

How to get to the heart of it. The key is to maintain intimacy, regardless of the role that sex plays. Intimacy will provide you both with a constant reminder that you're on the same team.

"He wonders how I can grieve so long"

What he might be trying to say or do: He may be unaware of how a loss can leave lasting effects on a woman, and want to understand the unique emotions that you have because the pregnancy took place in your body. You may feel connection, powerlessness, or guilt in totally different measures than he, and for much longer than he, simply because he was never responsible for safe carriage of the pregnancy.

How it can be taken badly: When our partner questions our grief it can seem callous and accusatory, as though we are fantasizing about something that never existed, or obsessing about something trivial.

How to get to the heart of it. Your feelings are legitimate, and accepting them is an important part of the healing process. If you can help your husband understand how the miscarriage has touched you then he will be better able to support you.

"He acts like I'm a hypochondriac because I want answers"

What he might be trying to say or do: He might want to know how investigation will help you. Many women report that following an intuition on testing or treatment worked out well for them in the end. If you are acting on your intuition, your partner may be struggling to understand.

How it can be taken badly: It can seem as if your partner is questioning your right to answers about your own body or your loss. In a situation where you may already feel powerless, having a partner who seems to be demanding justification can demoralize you further.

How to get to the heart of it. Talk to him about how taking action or getting answers will help you physically or mentally. Explore how he sees this situation as different from any other involving health concerns. (For example, if you found a lump in your breast, wouldn't prompt investigation yield the greatest benefits?)

Supporting each other

Maintaining a strong partnership requires that you continue acting as partners. Communication and intimacy are the key ingredients to a strong partnership, and the better you are at these the stronger the partnership will be. (Please note that "better" does not necessarily mean "more." For example, better communication might be achieved by knowing when not to talk about something – when it is time to give it a rest, leave something unsaid, or change the subject.)

Communication

Talking is generally a good thing, especially if it's done in a way that seeks to strengthen your team. For example, discussing the different ways in which the miscarriage impacted you can help you understand each other better, while blurting "Don't come near me with that thing!" in the bedroom is best avoided unless you have flawless Mae West delivery and a husband with an excellent sense of humor.

If communication is difficult, do not hesitate to seek help. Many people find it difficult to verbalize their feelings about painful or emotional subjects, and doing so can be scary, especially at the beginning. Working with a counselor can help get communication flowing; even one or two sessions can give you both tools for communicating more easily in the future.

Intimacy

This is the fun part, because it ranges from yoga to comedy to sex (or all three at once, if you can manage). Intimacy is built on mutual love, respect, and trust. It is created and maintained when you strengthen your bond; this comes from doing things that remind you of what you love about each other. Some ways of building intimacy are through:

Activities. Activities you both enjoy and do together are excellent. Of particular benefit are activities that let you laugh or relax (like comedy clubs or yoga classes), or that force you to be completely in the moment (like rock climbing or a challenging cooking class).

Some couples enjoy heated matches of ping pong, bowling, or board games; others enjoy working together on home improvement projects. The only important thing is that activities make you feel stronger as a team.

Special time. The demands of today's high-pressure, multi-tasking world can chisel away at the time we spend alone with our partners. Work, social commitments, and family responsibilities can all reduce the time we have to connect one-on-one.

Of course, none of those other things will benefit your long-term happiness as much as a good marriage will, and carving out some time for yourselves as a couple is a great investment.

Special time should be fun so that you look forward to it and enjoy being together; it should be frequent (once a week is a good guideline) and regular (e.g. every Thursday night) so that other commitments can be scheduled around it, giving it the priority it deserves. Special time should enable you to talk freely, and is best enjoyed away from home's distractions.

Gestures. Gestures should be given generously, as they are a sign to show you care. A gesture can be simple and spontaneous, like a note, a hug, or a phone call, or it can be bigger or more involved, like a special gift or a banner across the front of the house. The idea of a gesture is that it is a reminder of why or how much you love the other person.

Sex. While sex is undoubtedly a good way to demonstrate how much you love each other, if one person is hesitant to resume lovemaking after a miscarriage then this does not need to compromise intimacy. There are many other ways of creating and strengthening the special bonds of a couple, and if they are used well then intimacy should continue to thrive.

What more you can do

The more you can support your partner, the more that investment is likely to strengthen the bond between you. You can help him identify some of the conflicting pressures he might feel, talk openly with you about his feelings, and build a support network:

Identify feelings. Many men lack practice in identifying what they are feeling, and in accepting those feelings as legitimate and normal. Plus, it often seems easier to ignore painful feelings than to face them. But psychological well-being is more quickly achieved by those who acknowledge and accept the emotions they feel.

Encourage dialogue. Just as your partner is naturally positioned to be your greatest support, you are positioned to be his. If you can get him to talk to you about what he is feeling, you will both benefit, not only because you will understand him better, but because you will be helping provide the support that is so crucial to getting through this difficult time.

Build a support group. While men have friends, they rarely have a support network to turn to in the event of something as intimate as a miscarriage. You can help your partner by encouraging him to think about his own needs for support, and where that support might come from. Whether he gets it from a friend, a professional counselor, or a friendly bartender is of less importance than that he can speak frankly about issues important to him.

Summary

The fact of the matter is that you got into this difficult place together, and while it may be challenging at times, you can get through it together, too. The good news is that many couples report that a miscarriage strengthens their partnership in many ways.

The key, then, is to ensure that you are among the couples who come out better on the other side. While the balance of give and take will be different for each couple, there will need to be generous helpings of patience, trust, understanding and love given by both you and your partner.

The many tools that have been discussed in this chapter can help keep the bonds between you strong; anything that keeps your relationship thriving will ensure that the support you are giving and receiving is as constant and powerful as it can be.

understand your doctor

Jennifer's story

I turned 34 on our honeymoon, and between the ages of 34 and 40 I experienced seven pregnancy losses. Before that I had never had any health issues at all – I'd always been really healthy. Tests never determined a specific medical problem, but our desire to have a baby drove us to explore many doctors and clinics. Our experience was confusing, but ultimately successful.

Opinions on my medical records varied widely, and the doctors themselves were very different. One doctor seemed too passive, while another seemed too slick. One doctor convinced me to enter an experimental immunological therapy, while months later two other well-respected specialists advised me to stop the treatments immediately, saying they could compromise my immune system. Yet another physician strongly urged us to give up and enter an egg donor program after our first attempt at IVF failed. It was even suggested to my husband that he might be carrying a "funny gene" that could be leading to repeat miscarriages. How were we to decide who was right, especially in our increasingly desperate state?

Each time I miscarried I tried to have the attitude that it was my body telling me the pregnancy was wrong, and I determined to just go on until the pregnancy was right. I thought it was a streak of bad luck, but that I was going to beat the odds. I was going to keep going until I had my kids, and it became an emotional crusade in defiance of the message that I couldn't. I just kept at it.

Finally, we settled in with a physician from a well-reputed clinic. He was thoughtful, addressed our questions directly, and seemed "simpatico" with us. Under his clinic's close and highly professional supervision, our next IVF cycle was successful. Saskia was born just before my 40th birthday, followed by Annelise when I was 43.

Looking back, I think it is critical to meet with more than one clinic – and all doctors associated with it – in order to find the right fit. It isn't only credentials and success rates that matter – personal style is important, too. So much seems to be loose science that I think a lot of it comes down to the intuition of the physician.

If I had it to do over again, I would try to be more intuitive about the physicians, and move along faster on a personality basis. I would research the clinics more thoroughly, and gather more word-of-mouth input from others. It became clear once I made open enquiries which was the best clinic. You've got to talk to other women.

Also, having experienced the varied interpretations of test results, as well as multiple clinics and doctors, I think it's important to take charge of your medical record and follow your instincts. Do your homework, ask questions and demand answers. If something doesn't feel right, don't become a victim to it. Be informed. I've had friends do everything to beat the odds, and most get there somehow.

understand your doctor

The third member of our core group is our doctor. Although few of us would ask our doctor to dictate our family planning, he can end up having a huge influence on these very decisions. While this can be a positive if your doctor is someone with the same goals and priorities as you, this happy result is only possible if you create and cultivate it.

However, if you are like me, you may feel inexplicably intimidated when you step into a doctor's office.

Sure, doctors are busy. But they are there to help us. They *want* to help us. So why do so many of us go all shy? How do we make ourselves communicate our questions, concerns and ideas so that we can get the answers we need? How do we build a partnership? The rest of this chapter will help answer these questions.

Stepping into your doctor's shoes

Doctors chose a difficult, demanding medical career to learn how to help people. Their days are focused on identifying and meeting the needs of other people, and they think about their patients and puzzle through their problems long after they have left the office for the day.

A doctor is not free to decide whom he will see each day; nor can he choose patients the way patients choose doctors. He does not have the option of asking around to determine your background and training, or to find out whether you're a "good" or "recommended" patient before agreeing to see you, the way you can with him. And he is unlikely to replace patients with whom he does not feel a bond, while patients can replace him whenever they like.

And although the doctor can tell a patient the way he thinks best to proceed, he cannot make her take medicine, change her lifestyle, or even keep her doctor's appointments. While a doctor might see the way forward very clearly, his patient might flatly refuse to believe it or try it. Surprisingly, the patient holds most of the power.

Of course, despite their exterior professionalism, most doctors are sensitive and empathetic, which is what led them into medicine in the first place. So they can sense unease or mistrust. As one doctor explained, "You can tell when someone doesn't like you, and it's awful. No matter what you do, they're going to be critical. Of course, with that kind of pressure, you *do* make more mistakes."

On the flip side, another doctor explained that when interaction is easy and natural, he is more likely to pick up on small, even subliminal clues about the problem that he might otherwise have missed. The sense of trust and connection sparks his intuition and creativity, skills which cannot be summoned under pressure.

So why are so many of us intimidated by these kind, educated, humanitarian people? Perhaps it's because we sometimes forget that they *are* people. And like all people, they will have totally unique ways of interacting, explaining things, and approaching problems. They might be relaxed or alarmist, cold or cuddly, intense or distracted, enthusiastic about experimental therapies or distrustful of them. All they have in common is that they want to help people.

But that doesn't mean that every doctor would be right for you.

How do you feel about medical authority?

Some people believe medical science is infallible; others think that even seeing a doctor is unlucky. Still others believe investigation is typically inconclusive, and therefore a waste of time and money. Some people shy away from discussing their concerns with medical staff, afraid they will appear stupid by asking a question, or that they may not understand the answer. However you look at it, most of us approach the medical profession with some intimidation. And naturally we tend to shy away from situations we find intimidating.

If you have a strong aversion to medical personnel or testing, this will influence how you interact with your doctor. Clarifying how comfortable you are in the face of medical expertise can help you address areas of concern, and the questionnaire below is designed to help you do this.

Self-assessment: how do you feel about medical authority?

(Tick the box for Yes)

1. *The information medical exams yield is usually useful, reliable, and conclusive* ☐
2. *The medical profession will not treat me impersonally or make me feel small* ☐
3. *It is possible that in certain cases I could know more about a medical issue or advance than a doctor* ☐
4. *I generally get good value when I see a doctor or have medical tests done* ☐
5. *I believe my questions and concerns are legitimate, and expect medical professionals to answer them* ☐
6. *Going to the doctor makes me less likely to have serious health problems in the future* ☐
7. *Even if medical tests found a problem I would see that as good, because then I could do something about it* ☐

Total Yes Answers: ☐

Interpreting the results

Score: 0-1

You are not at all comfortable with medical professionals, and try to avoid them. This is likely to hamper your ability to get answers when you need them, and to form a partnership with your doctor.

Score: 2-4

You probably find medical exams embarrassing or awkward, or may dislike asking questions of medical professionals. These misgivings will make you shy away from any "non-essential" interaction with your doctor, and will make forming a partnership more challenging.

Score: 5-7

You are prepared to ask questions about what you think is important, and to try to understand medical issues relevant to you. This attitude will help you create a solid working relationship with your doctor that is based on mutual respect.

Know the doctor you've got

Most of us don't choose a doctor based on mutual trust, respect, or affection, the way we choose a friend or partner. We find someone through word of mouth, history, or happenstance, and if they get the job done then they're good enough. But this is someone who may tell you the happiest or saddest news of your life, and with whom you will share your life's most significant moments; this person should be chosen with care.

My own doctor had a busy practice and a full waiting room. I called him "Doctor" and he called me "Susan." I could never bring myself to call him "Bob." He wasn't that kind of guy.

His elderly receptionist weighed all patients in the waiting room, repeating their weight loudly over and over as she shuffled back to her desk. But by the time she got there she had to shout out, "What was it again, love?" and the mortified patient had to call out her weight.

The doctor himself was no more sensitive. With each of my miscarriages the only comfort he offered was by way of saying, "You just have very bad luck," followed by, "So you shouldn't be wasting your time on research. Just go home and forget it ever happened. Try again. That's all you can do." He told me that six times.

So why was his waiting room full? Perhaps because we tend to think it is too hard to change to a new doctor when we're already heavily invested in another. To avoid staying with a doctor you don't want, it is important to evaluate the doctor you've got.

Evaluating your relationship with your doctor

In your own relationship with your doctor, do you feel there is a good, solid rapport between you? Could your interactions be improved? Is the situation beyond help? The questionnaire below may help you answer some of these questions.

Self-assessment: how "simpatico" is your doctor?

(Tick the box for Yes)

1. *I believe my doctor is up-to-date on the issues and advances relevant to my situation* ☐
2. *My doctor has had many patients like me, yet treats me as an individual* ☐
3. *My doctor and I would likely agree on whether and when testing is right, and how broad it should be* ☐
4. *I think my doctor and I would probably have the same ideas about what treatments were appropriate for me* ☐
5. *I feel I can ask my doctor about anything that concerns me and he would be happy to explain it thoroughly* ☐
6. *My doctor takes my concerns as seriously as I do* ☐
7. *When I ask my doctor questions he does not take them as an affront to his authority or a waste of his time* ☐

Total Yes Answers: ☐

Interpreting the results

Score: 0-2

You and your doctor lack the rapport that can be so comforting. Difficulties are so extensive that it may be more productive for you to replace your doctor rather than try to fix the relationship.

Score: 3-5

You probably have a cordial working relationship with your doctor, but do not see him or her as a part of your team. Depending upon the difficulties, you may be able to improve your relationship, or you may decide it is better to find another doctor.

Score: 6-7

You enjoy an excellent relationship with your doctor, and see him as a positive member of your team. You probably already do most of the things discussed below in "Working Well With Your Doctor," and are reaping the rewards of doing so.

Working well with your doctor

A good relationship with a doctor is like any good relationship – it works best when based on mutual respect, trust, and personality fit:

Mutual respect

This is a two-way street, and problems can arise on either side. You may respect your doctor, but feel he doesn't take your concerns seriously. Or your doctor may be capable and professional, but you are not convinced of his ability to offer you the expertise you need or the range of options you might want.

Your respect for your doctor

If you doubt your doctor's training or expertise then this is a serious problem. If this is simply because you are unsure of his qualifications, then following the tips below may resolve this uncertainty. But if your confidence has faltered because of something he did (or failed to do), then this is a more challenging problem. Your options are to do nothing and continue worrying about the quality of care you are getting, speak to your doctor and broach the delicate subject of his expertise or approach, or change doctors and build a new relationship. Obviously, none of these is easy to do.

Tips for promoting respect for your doctor

The more you know about your doctor, the more likely you are to find common ground. The information below can usually be gleaned from the Internet or a "new patient" call to the doctor's office.

Find out about your doctor's training and experience. Where and when did your doctor do his medical training? How long has he been in practice? Does he have a particular specialty area? If he has not been at this practice for long, what did he do prior?

Explore the capabilities of his practice. What resources does the practice offer? What specialists are on hand? What does the practice think it does well?

Determine if he has other interests or achievements. Has your doctor written articles or research reports on an area of particular interest? Has he been involved with worthwhile community projects? Does he have other areas of interest or achievement?

Get to know him. Your doctor is one of your most intimate relationships, and is therefore worth knowing better. Chat with him as you would anyone with whom you have a close relationship. Why did he choose this particular practice or specialty area? What were his motivations? Have they changed since he started in practice?

Listen to what he says. Listening carefully to what your doctor says will give you a good sense of how he thinks and what his priorities are. This will help you anticipate areas where your natural preferences might diverge, and facilitate constructive discussions.

Your doctor's respect for you

Your doctor's respect for you will dictate how readily he seeks your input when planning your healthcare. Do not confuse professionalism with respect, as I did. My doctor was always professional, and because I mistook this for respect, I failed to act on many signs that he did not want my input.

Tips for promoting your doctor's respect for you

Treat him with respect. Always treat your doctor as a respected professional, even if you disagree with his approach or style. His desire to help people was strong enough to sustain him through the rigors of medical training; it is unlikely that his goal is to intimidate or aggravate you! Imagine him as a respected colleague. How would you phrase questions, and what style of response would you expect?

Communicate with him. Try to have frank conversations about things that concern you. For example, when my doctor said testing was not worth it, I should have asked why. I would have learned that he thought it best for a woman if she pretended a miscarriage had never happened. I could have explained that, in my case, not having answers would prevent me from putting the issue to rest. Those mutual insights would have helped us clarify what was best for me.

Let him know the role you intend to play in your own healthcare. Even if your doctor perfectly understands your point of view, this does not mean he has to agree with you. It is what happens from there that makes the difference between a strong partnership and a bad experience. A doctor should be prepared to present a variety of options, their pros and cons, and his own recommendations, all the while working in conjunction with you. It is not his role – and probably not his desire – to take responsibility for your healthcare.

Give him all the information he needs. You need to communicate everything that might be relevant, so try to have actual dates and specific details handy. Telling him you had an abortion at eight weeks gestation when you were 19, and that your current pregnancy took 18 months to achieve is of much more use than leaving those details out, or a vague reference to "some trouble" with pregnancy.

Be a good patient. A "good patient" is not the same as a "good girl." A good patient is one who is informed and knowledgeable, who answers questions as specifically as possible, and who asks questions in a way that is not confrontational. For example, "Why didn't you order this certain test?" probably won't give you much useful information. Asking, "Can you tell me about the tests you're ordering, and what you're hoping to find out from them?" gives you the chance to learn about how your doctor thinks. Once you've listened to his answer, you might say, "I thought this certain test would be a good one for me. Have you considered it?" and again listen to his answer. The idea is not to win points in a debate, but rather to effectively manage your healthcare; doctors are crucial to helping you do so.

Trust

Like any good relationship, trust plays a crucial role in the bond you have with your doctor. The level of trust you have in him comes down to how strongly you believe he will do what is best for you.

Of course, to do what is best for you, your doctor has to balance his medical experience with your personal preferences. For example, he might be convinced that your best chance of successful pregnancy is through IVF, but if you do not want to pursue that course then he needs to support your decision by helping you evaluate other options.

Tips for building trust with your doctor

Communicate your priorities. Without knowing your goals, your doctor can only make recommendations based on past experience with other patients. While this may work well most of the time, it may not always fit your unique preferences. If you are concerned about a course of action, or want more information before making a decision, then discussing these issues with your doctor is a must.

Create effective roles. People often play the roles others expect them to play. So if you want your doctor to be part of your team, acting that way will make it easier for him to work in partnership with you.

Personality fit

Of course, the most serious problem with my doctor was that he had a whole different approach than I did; we had no personality fit. His approach was to "keep trying, and eventually you'll get there." With my 10% chance of success, he was technically correct. It's just that I didn't want to have nine miscarriages for every baby I delivered.

So the question is: is your doctor of the same profile as you? Does he seem to take things as seriously as you do? If not, does he have a satisfactory explanation (i.e. solid medical evidence that pertains to you, not just statistics) as to why this lack of concern is appropriate in your case? If there is not a good fit, you run the risk of a destructive clash if the going gets tough.

Replacing a doctor

Sometimes no amount of working on a relationship will fix it, and this is no less true with doctors than with anyone else. While replacing a doctor provokes a lot of uncertainty, it is also an opportunity to start fresh with someone who might ultimately have a very positive influence on your life.

So how do you do it? It all comes down to research and evaluation.

Research

Before determining whether or not a doctor may be right for you, you need to find out who those doctors might be. Finding those names is the result of research conducted through a variety of sources:

Network of contacts

This is where most people start, as family, friends and colleagues are easy to approach, happy to help, and good sources of firsthand experience.

Your female friends and colleagues are likely to have much in common with you, and their impressions may be similar to yours; if they found a doctor kind, responsive, and well-informed, then you might feel the same way. When speaking to them make sure to find out exactly what they like about the doctor they are recommending.

Doctor recommendations

Your GP (general practitioner), if you have one, will be able to recommend a few obstetrician-gynecologists, and if you have a good working relationship with your GP then you might enjoy the same kind of relationship with someone he recommends.

Getting recommendations from doctors other than your GP can be more of a challenge, but it can be done. For example, a colleague of mine contacted five female obstetrician-gynecologists that had been recommended to her, and somehow found out who they had chosen as their own doctors when they were pregnant. Finding that four of the five had used the same doctor, she knew she'd found her new doctor.

Your insurance company

Your insurance company may have a list of doctors in your area that they work with. While this will give you a database of names, you will need to research them further to determine their suitability.

Medical associations

There are medical associations in almost every county and state in the US, as well as the American Medical Association (AMA) which covers the whole country. These associations are typically staffed and run by doctors, and their goal is to improve medical care. A doctor doesn't have to be a member of any association, but most are, as they receive a number of benefits such as news of relevant medical developments and inclusion on referral lists.

Medical associations keep lists of doctors sorted geographically and by practice specialty. Practice areas relevant to pregnancy are: general practice (GP), family medicine, obstetrics & gynecology, and reproductive medicine (or fertility specialists).

The AMA website provides a DoctorFinder service, and says that it has "virtually every licensed physician in the United States" in its database. Many of them are not AMA members, however, and only their most basic information is provided (name, specialty, city of practice, and telephone number). Many doctors choose not to be a member of the AMA, but are instead a member of their county or state association, considering the information and referrals more local and relevant. Thus, state or county medical associations may be able to provide more detailed listings for many doctors.

Through these channels you can often get good information about a doctor's training and credentials. In addition, medical associations record whether a doctor has any judgments against him (cases of malpractice or negligence); if your doctor is not a member of any medical association, it is worth asking why.

The Internet

Without fairly specific search criteria, getting information off the Internet can be like trying to get a glass of water out of a fire hose.

If you are simply trying to find doctors practicing in your city, the Internet may have too much information. If, however, you have specific requirements or questions, the Internet can be an excellent resource. For example, if you need a particular kind of reproductive specialist, the Internet can be an effective way of identifying options. Similarly, if you already have a list of potential doctors, and want to find out more information about them, then the Internet may provide a wealth of such information.

Evaluation

Ask the questions

Once you have narrowed down your list to a manageable number, call the offices of your top candidates and ask questions that will help you make a final decision. These may include such questions as:

- How do I become a patient? Do I need a referral? How long after conception should I call in order to be assured a place?
- How far into pregnancy is the first consultation? Does this depend on my history? (If you have had a loss and the doctor will not see you until 10 weeks, he may not be right for you.)
- What do patients say about his bedside manner? Is he a good listener? Does he take time to explain things to patients?
- How regularly and reliably does the doctor return patient's calls?
- How quickly could I get an appointment if a problem arose?
- What are the doctor's fees for consultation?
- What is his consultation schedule during pregnancy? (e.g. once a month until 30-32 weeks, then every two weeks ...)
- At what hospital would the birth take place? (If you want "non-standard" birthing options, like a home birth or an elective caesarian section, this may be the time to mention it.)
- In the event the birth or complications occur after-hours, does the doctor attend, or does he "rotate" with other doctors? Who are the other doctors, and do patients get to meet them prior to labor?
- What are his success rates (if he is a specialist)?

These are too many questions to ask a busy receptionist. However, she should be willing to spend a few minutes on the phone with you, or suggest a more convenient time to call back. If the receptionist is very busy but wants to help you, then calling back is worthwhile. But if she is difficult or uninformed then it may not be the right place for you, as she will be the one fielding your call in an emergency.

Get on the list

Many women are unpleasantly surprised when they try to make an appointment only a week or two after their first missed period and find that a doctor's practice is already full. Especially if you are a new patient, it is important to call for an appointment as soon as you know you are pregnant, as this gets you on the doctor's list. The appointment itself might be weeks away, but getting in early ensures you do not miss out.

You may want to consider making appointments with the two or three doctors that appeal most to you, so that you can meet them and decide which you prefer.

Make a decision

If you see your top choice doctor first, you may be able to save yourself the time and expense of going to a second or third doctor. However, if you have any reservations about the first doctor you see, then it is probably worth the extra expense of going to the next. While appointments can be expensive, it can be a good investment if you end up with a doctor you are very happy with. Had I done that with my first doctor I may have spared myself years of frustration and avoided several miscarriages.

The first appointment

After all you have done to research and choose your new doctor, you will want your first appointment to be as productive as possible. It is important that your new doctor get a thorough understanding of your relevant medical history, goals, and priorities. You should bring:

- Copies of your medical records from other doctors or clinics.
- A summary sheet of relevant gynecological history. Particularly if you have had difficulty with conception, complications in pregnancy, or losses, it is important to give your doctor all the details. You do not need to give him the sheet, but you need to ensure he knows everything on it. If any tests were done then bring copies of the results.
- Your partner (or someone else) for moral support if it will help you relax and get through everything. Do not bring children or anyone that will distract you or the doctor, make it difficult to talk openly about your history, or require you to interrupt the appointment. This is an important session for you and the doctor to get to know each other, and the more positive and productive it can be, the better for everyone.

Traversing common pitfalls

If you are worried that you may be at higher risk of miscarriage, then it can be quite difficult to decide what you want to do. Communicating your decisions to a doctor who has different plans can be even harder. In miscarriage assessment, the most frequent subjects of disagreement are testing and treatment. Below are some common points on which doctors and patients disagree, and some ways of addressing these issues.

When is the right time to investigate miscarriage?

In the past, many doctors refused to test for miscarriage causes before a woman had suffered three miscarriages in a row. However, because two miscarriages already indicate a greater risk of having another, the American College of Obstetrics and Gynecologists now recommends testing after a second loss, particularly for women over the age of 35. This is good to know if you want early testing.

Is testing worth it?

Many doctors will argue that testing is not worth it. However, many women feel that using their pregnancies as "tests" in order to save the time, money, or physical discomfort associated with lab exams is a much higher price to pay. For them it is worth it to do everything possible to avoid more miscarriages.

Aside from the psychological benefits associated with testing, some medical practitioners are beginning to realize that testing makes financial sense as well. For example, while chromosomal analysis of miscarried tissue can cost $400-$600, it can help focus further work. If it comes out abnormal then that explains the miscarriage and there is no need for further testing, which can cost several thousand dollars.

How much testing or treatment is "appropriate"?

How much testing or treatment you're comfortable with is something only you can decide. While your doctor will make recommendations based on his experience and insights into your own case, you are the one that is going to have to live with it. Only you can say whether a particular test or procedure is what you want at this particular time. Your doctor may be a valued advisor in this situation, but it is not up to him to decide whether you should undergo IVF, or experimental immunotherapy, or anything. All those decisions should be yours, because you have to live with them.

Your doctor is a highly trained expert in his field, and while you have paid for his advice, you are not obligated to take it. If you want second opinions or further information, you are completely within your rights to seek them. In the end, it's up to you.

Summary

Your doctor plays a key role in your life, not only because he can help you identify the best healthcare options for your unique circumstances, but also because he will be part of some of your most intimate moments. How confident you feel in pregnancy, and how empowered you feel about yourself, can hinge on your relationship with your doctor, so it is worth cultivating a relationship characterized by mutual respect, trust, and good personality fit.

looking toward the future

choosing your own path

Helen's story

We started trying to get pregnant when I was 29, but were unable to. We had all the tests, which came back normal. Although I had a history of endometriosis, doctors said it didn't play a part in the difficulty we were having. I hated that they couldn't find a cause, because I wanted to do something. But of course you can't fix a problem you can't find.

Four years after we'd started trying to conceive, we turned to IVF. We were very lucky because I conceived on the very first IVF cycle, and Phoebe was born at full term, happy and healthy.

Ten months later I felt really tired. We weren't using any birth control, but after all the trouble we'd had getting pregnant I thought it was impossible I'd get pregnant unintentionally. Plus, I was still breastfeeding and hadn't had a period yet. We were absolutely astonished to find out I was 14 weeks pregnant!

We'd always wanted three children, and 10 months after Ella was born I was pregnant for the third time. At 11 weeks I had spotting – no pain, but enough blood to make me go see my doctor. Because I'd had a lot of blood loss with my other two pregnancies I didn't think it had to be a miscarriage, but a scan showed an empty pregnancy sac. I opted to have a D&C, but decided against karyotyping, as I didn't think it was necessary. I was convinced it was a genetic problem, and not meant to be.

The doctors who managed my miscarriage said that if I didn't get pregnant again within six months I should go back to the IVF clinic, so I did.

The IVF people didn't want to investigate any further, and my first consultation was bad. The doctor looked at my history and my age (I was 35) and told me, "If you go ahead without IVF, it's my opinion you have less than a 1% chance of becoming pregnant." Then he took out his calendar, asked where I was in my cycle, and started looking at dates. He just assumed I would be doing IVF, as though that were that. I could so easily have lost control of events! I was disappointed because I felt he was selling me a plan of action I didn't really need, without considering how it would change my life.

I had a lot of emotions about the whole thing. I'm a control freak, so the complete lack of control I had experienced through the whole process was very challenging for me to deal with. Plus, I was genuinely disappointed that we wouldn't have a third child. But at the same time I was very grateful that we were a family of four.

I found that the comments people make, not meaning to be unkind, can be very hurtful. Questions like "When are you going to have children and stop focusing on your career?" as we were experiencing infertility, or "Why on earth would you be considering IVF when you've got two children?" I know people don't mean to be nasty, but you're trying to deal with so much. I had to keep telling myself, "Just relax – you're too stressed."

My husband and I wanted to work to our own plan, and felt that we were already blessed with two children. We decided not to go down the IVF track, and to continue trying on our own. Six months later I was pregnant with Thomas, and when he was born our family was complete.

My experience convinced me how important it is to be really proactive about the choices you make – to be informed about all the options, and not to be afraid to ask for a second opinion. That approach let us choose the path that was right for us by being in partnership with my doctors, making informed decisions, and being involved in the outcome we achieved. That made all the difference in how I felt, and in how things turned out for us.

choosing your own path

By picking up this book you have already taken positive action for your future. You may decide that you do not need to go any further than this book, as that is the right decision for you. Or you may decide to vigorously pursue additional information, as that is appropriate for you. Whatever decision you make must be based upon your own needs, priorities, and preferences, because only then it will be right for you.

This chapter is designed to help you determine the course of action that is right for you.

Inner strength

I have been amazed by the women who shared their stories with me. These women had to grapple with the loss of a child they had already seen in their imagination. And they spoke of many other things they had lost: their innocent wonder for future pregnancies; their feelings of youthful invincibility; even their sense of power or purpose.

While each of them had to weather a loss (or many losses), the extraordinary thing was that when they told me their stories, they each mentioned something positive. They might have talked about how their husband had supported them and how that had ultimately brought them closer, or how they realized that by having confidence in their own judgment they could find their own solution, or even the satisfaction that comes from having a child after you've been told you never will. These women had each managed to take something positive from their ordeals.

So how do you summon your strength and courage and direct it into positive action? By clarifying what it is you want, and the best options for achieving it.

Your plan

The women I interviewed remained focused on their goal, and felt sustained by the strength of their own resolve, their husbands, and/or their doctors.

While few women stated that they had a specific plan, they all had a clear goal, whether it was "To just keep trying until I had my kids," "To pursue every available avenue," or "To learn everything I could about how to beat my problem, and then do it." Each of these statements is a plan. Every woman had a clear vision of what she wanted to achieve, and some idea of ways to get there. Of course, the goals were often short-term, and subject to change so that they served the women, rather than the other way around.

Having read through this book, you now have a solid understanding of miscarriage causes and treatments, a good idea of your own risk profile, and insights into the kind of information and support you need. You have thought about your near-term goals, and the constraints you need to address in order to achieve them.

All that is left is to consolidate it into a simple plan that will put you on the path you want to be on, and take you in the direction you want to go.

The general direction

In the chapter *Understand Yourself* you considered pressures that might impact the path you choose. But if you know your own mind it is easier to meet your own needs within the constraints of your circumstances.

Therefore, in order to see what you, in your heart of hearts, would really like to do, imagine for the next (and final) questionnaire that you have all the time, money, and support that you want.

self-assessment: general direction

(Tick the box for Yes)

1. *I want answers about my own miscarriage risk profile that I can get only from medical professionals or tests* ☐
2. *Medical evaluation would help my peace of mind* ☐
3. *I'd like a medical investigation to see if there are any problems with my carrying a pregnancy to term* ☐
4. *I can't be confident or comfortable in my next pregnancy without concrete medical results* ☐
5. *I don't want to get pregnant and "wait and see" if it works without first doing a medical investigation* ☐
6. *I want to learn whatever I can from a previous pregnancy loss so it isn't "wasted"* ☐
7. *Getting answers will help me regain control of my life* ☐

Total Yes Answers: ☐

Interpreting the results

Score: 0-1 *(general direction: relaxed but alert)*

Either you are fairly confident of the success of future pregnancies, or feel you can get the information you need from resources like this book. Women who choose this general direction will stay alert to miscarriage, but do not feel the need to take any medical action before going on to future pregnancies.

Score: 2-4 *(general direction: address areas of specific interest)*

Women who choose this general direction do not feel they need a full medical investigation. However, they may have specific areas of concern they want to know more about or investigate further. This may mean doing more research, discussing the issue with a specialist, or having testing in the specific area of concern.

Score: 5-7 *(general direction: maximum information)*

Women who choose this general direction want solid answers and are willing to take action to maximize their chance of successful pregnancy. If there were no constraining factors to consider, these women would likely do whatever they could to get maximum information before going ahead with further pregnancies.

The specific plan

Once you've identified your general direction, formulating a specific plan does not have to be a daunting exercise. A plan can be written down or merely considered, sketchy or comprehensive, for the long-term or just for now. The only important thing is that your plan reflect what is best for you. Some examples of simple plans include:

- We will go on as before
- We will get testing (comprehensive, or in areas of specific concern)
- We will see what the next pregnancy brings and then reevaluate
- I will develop an excellent support network before becoming pregnant again
- I will change my doctor
- I will consult a specialist
- We will investigate whether IVF can increase our chance of healthy pregnancy
- I will explore other options (e.g. herbal remedies)
- We are ready for closure, and will not try again

Because you are more likely to complete your plan if you keep it simple, you may want to limit it to one or two steps. Once one plan has been accomplished, it is easy and gratifying to create another. Conversely, any plan is likely to appear impossible if it is too complicated or carried out too far into the future.

Maintaining perspective

Once you have chosen your plan, you are on a path toward your goal. Of course, as with any path, there are likely to be unforeseen events or setbacks along the way. For example, a medical investigation that finds nothing wrong may seem to be a waste of time and money. But women with this information are usually more confident with their next pregnancy than if they had lingering doubts about their ability to carry a baby to term, and the studies mentioned in *The Power of Love* indicate that their chance of success is as high as 86% with the right support. For women whose medical investigations do find a problem, they have a better chance of getting effective treatment and having a successful pregnancy the next time.

Also, deciding to stop trying and get on with the rest of your life requires just as much courage – or more – as continuing. For couples that have invested a great deal in trying to have a baby, this can be a wrenching decision. However, many couples report feeling relieved and liberated when they decide to move on. Only you can determine whether you have pursued all the options you want to, and whether you will regret not trying once more.

What if treatment fails?

Many treatments have high success rates for subsequent pregnancy. But while success rates of 75-80% are impressive odds, they still mean that one in every four to five pregnancies will end in a loss. What if pregnancy after treatment ends in miscarriage?

If you do suffer a loss after receiving treatment, then it was either because the pregnancy had a random, unrelated problem, or because your underlying condition was not adequately addressed:

Random chance. If your loss was due to a random error in the pregnancy, then your chances of carrying a baby to term the next time could still be as high as anyone's; it is essential to have the miscarriage analyzed to confirm whether it was indeed due to chance.

Underlying condition. If analysis confirms that the loss was not due to random chance, then your underlying condition was not adequately addressed. In that case, changing specialist or adjusting treatment might solve the problem. For example, you might improve your outlook by finding a clinic with a better record of success, or having your current specialist augment low-dose aspirin with heparin, or exploring whether you might have more than one underlying condition.

Summary

Whatever path you choose, so long as it is based on what you think is best for you, then it is the right path for you. Being convinced of this will help you overcome any obstacles you may encounter. No one should try to talk you into taking a path you don't want, as no one else is as well-positioned as you are to determine what is best for you.

enjoying pregnancy

Tiffany's story

By the time I was pregnant for the third time (after having two easy, trouble-free pregnancies) I was very relaxed – almost blasé. We had just moved to a new city where my husband's family lived, and as I had to ask them to recommend a doctor, we shared news of our pregnancy at about five weeks. Shortly thereafter they announced our good news at a huge family reunion!

As a result, we had to tell our own children, and Eliza and Hixon then shared the news with their classes for show and tell! So by the time we were eight weeks along, about 200 people knew we were pregnant, even though I had only told five people myself!

At my first appointment with my doctor (at nine weeks) the ultrasound showed a mass that had stopped developing at five weeks. I started miscarrying the next day. When it got heavy I went to the emergency room, where I sat for seven hours in an uncomfortable plastic chair in the waiting room having a miscarriage. They only had one private room for internal exams, and someone else beat me to it. They finally examined me and did the D&C within 20 minutes.

Analysis of the D&C confirmed what they'd seen on ultrasound – it was never going to be a baby or have a heartbeat – it never organized itself.

I knew how common miscarriage was, and thought my chance of having one somewhere along the way was pretty high. It's just a numbers game – I thought that at 36 years of age a certain percentage of my eggs could be bad. I felt my miscarriage was just a bad egg. I wasn't upset so much as I was just surprised, since our previous pregnancies had been so uneventful.

I wasn't worried it would happen again (though I may have been more concerned if I had miscarried before having two kids!)

The midwife said, "There is absolutely no reason why you can't have another healthy baby. This happens all the time. Do not let this be of concern to you at all."

It was upsetting facing the family, and I cried a couple of times, but I didn't think it was tragic; I genuinely felt okay about it. I looked forward to my next pregnancy being easy and trouble-free, which it was. There were no problems – it was another really easy pregnancy – and it gave us our son Rockwood about 11 months after the miscarriage.

I think it's important to share both your pregnancy and your miscarriage with people who can support you. While having 200 people know about it was probably too many, that fluke of circumstances showed that the net can be wider than you think. People know you're going through something, and they cut you some slack; not telling them and dealing with it privately behind the scenes means you're acting in a weird way that they don't understand. If they know, then they're compassionate and supportive. Who's going to hold it against you? Did it matter that 200 people knew? No.

In fact, I feel like it brought me closer to some people. For example, my mother-in-law had two or three miscarriages after her first child was born, before going on to have four more children without any problem; we connected on a very personal level.

enjoying pregnancy

Pregnancy can be one of life's most exhilarating, empowering experiences. Or it can be fraught with confusion or anxiety. For many women, it is all of these things at once.

How, then, to enjoy pregnancy as much as possible, especially if you are concerned?

There are several things you can do to make your pregnancy more enjoyable, many of which may even give you a higher chance of success. Essentially, good health and a strong body, combined with a comfortable emotional state of mind, will pay great dividends.

Prepare for pregnancy

It is always easier to enjoy something if we are happy and relaxed. So the more you can prepare for pregnancy, and do things that will help you approach your next pregnancy with more confidence, the more likely you are to enjoy it.

For example, if you want to have tests or immunizations to increase your peace of mind (such as for Chickenpox or toxoplasmosis), then this is the time to do so. If you want to change your doctor, then now is the time to do the research, make the decision, and put the change in place. If you want to undertake a cleansing diet prior to becoming pregnant, follow a herbalist's advice to prepare your body for healthy pregnancy, get in better physical or psychological condition prior to conception, or taper off a grueling training regimen before becoming pregnant, then achieving these things in advance of pregnancy can help you feel empowered and prepared for a good experience.

While your own preparations will be unique, as they are based upon your own situation, some things to consider include:

Getting answers. If having more information on issues that concern you will help you feel more confident in your next pregnancy, then getting that information should be a top priority.

If you are hesitant to pursue answers because you worry that it might show there is something wrong, remember that a risk can only be overcome once it has been identified. Not knowing about an underlying condition does not make your miscarriage risk go away, it simply means you do not have the tools to address that risk.

Cultivating your support group. In addition to increasing your personal fulfillment, extra care and support have been linked to improved pregnancy outcome, as discussed in *The Power of Love*; now is the time to strengthen your own support. The ideal support group is composed of people who can help you throughout pregnancy, supporting you through times of anxiety and celebrating with you in times of joy.

Choosing a doctor or specialist. Identify whom you would like to be your doctor during pregnancy, and put any necessary groundwork in place (e.g. paperwork, initial consultation, etc).

Having a check-up. To determine your immunity to rubella, Chickenpox, toxoplasmosis, measles, mumps, etc. If you find you are susceptible to any of these, immunizations are available for almost all of them.

Screening for infection. You may want to test for vaginal or uterine infection that could jeopardize a pregnancy. If an infection is present, there is likely effective treatment; for infections that can't be treated there are steps you can take to protect your pregnancy.

Planning your health management. If you have any conditions that require close management during pregnancy (such as diabetes), have a discussion with your doctor about any strategies you need to put in place.

Reviewing lifestyle modification. It is important to discuss with your doctor any diet or exercise modification you may be considering prior to, or during, pregnancy.

Living healthy. Healthy eating habits and regular moderate-intensity exercise will benefit you before, during, and after pregnancy.

Reviewing medication. Discuss with your doctor any medication you may be taking, and find out how safe it is for conception and pregnancy.

Having dental work. Have dental appointments before you become pregnant, as x-rays or work you may need are best done then.

Taking supplements. Folic acid (also called "folate") supplements are an important part of preparing for pregnancy. Folate significantly reduces the incidence of spina bifida (an open spine, one of the most common birth defects). While folate is found in food such as spinach and berries, it is difficult to get it in the amounts required. A daily dose of 400µg beginning three months before conception and continuing through the end of the first trimester is considered ideal. Supplemental folic acid is available on its own or as an ingredient in most pregnancy supplements; check the label to confirm dosage.

Kicking the habit(s). Now is the time to stop smoking, drinking, or any other habits that could harm a pregnancy.

Cutting down on caffeine. Evaluate your caffeine intake and cut back if necessary, replacing regular tea with herbal tea, caffeinated coffee with decaf, caffeinated soft drinks with fruit juice or soft drinks containing no caffeine. Check the label on chocolate and energy drinks, which can have more caffeine than you'd expect.

Updating insurance coverage. Review your health insurance to determine what it does and does not cover, and make any necessary changes (there are often long "wait times" for pregnancy coverage, so changes should be made as soon as possible, and wait times should be clearly understood). Insurance companies vary widely in their coverage of reproductive healthcare, so be clear on your own policy's coverage and requirements.

The summary checklist on the following page may help you keep track of your preparations.

Summary checklist: preparing for pregnancy

- *Get answers to any issues of concern* ☐
- *Strengthen your support group* ☐
- *Choose a doctor or specialist* ☐
- *Have a pre-pregnancy check-up for immunity* ☐
- *Screen for infection that can harm pregnancy* ☐
- *Plan management of any chronic health issues* ☐
- *Review any diet or exercise plans with your doctor* ☐
- *Improve eating and exercise habits* ☐
- *Review your medications with your doctor* ☐
- *Have any dental work that you need done* ☐
- *Begin taking folic acid supplements* ☐
- *Kick any habit(s) that could harm a pregnancy* ☐
- *Cut down on caffeine* ☐
- *Update your insurance coverage* ☐

Enjoy it as it unfolds

Going through your next pregnancy with greater confidence will not only enable you to enjoy it more, it may even improve your chance of success. Read through the suggestions below to see which ones might help you enjoy the experience more fully.

Take care of yourself. Just as people might say you are "eating for two," you are caring for two. This does not mean it is your fault if something goes wrong; it simply means you are entitled to a great deal of tender loving care.

The women in the studies mentioned in *The Power of Love* were not only given increased medical and psychological care, they were advised to take two weeks off at the gestational age of their last loss, and to avoid strenuous work and travel. In short, they were advised to treat themselves more kindly. And they were repaid with an incredibly high pregnancy success rate.

It can sometimes be difficult to put yourself ahead of your professional or personal obligations. But your baby deserves a gentle touch, and you do too. While we have many demands in life that require us to prove how tough we are, pregnancy is one of the times we can show ourselves how much we matter, and how gently and kindly we can treat ourselves.

Feel healthy and strong. It is easier to feel confident and in control when we feel healthy and strong. Not only are we more physically robust, but this sense of power permeates our whole being, making us more resilient and increasing our ability to cope with the hurdles life throws in our way.

By increasing your resilience, a healthy body will also increase your enjoyment of pregnancy (and life, for that matter). The benefits extend not only to pre-pregnancy, but also throughout pregnancy and beyond, and are as diverse as lower rates of gestational diabetes, fewer muscle strains during and after pregnancy, and higher quality sleep.

Draw on your support group. A good support network will enhance all aspects of your life, and may be particularly beneficial to pregnancy. Do not hesitate to draw on your support group to share your experience with you.

Go alternative, if you like. What role do alternative therapies such as acupuncture, herbal remedies, and homeopathy have in all this? Whatever role you like.

Because so much about miscarriage is not yet understood, who can say that alternative therapies do not increase your odds of success? Of course, it is always a good idea to discuss your plans with your doctor. But if it is something that you want to pursue, and it makes you feel more relaxed, healthy, strong, empowered, or happy, then the support it provides is already of value.

Relax and lighten up. Pregnancy can be a difficult time to relax, as there are anxieties about the pregnancy, tasks to accomplish before the baby arrives, and too many uncertainties to even think about beyond that. Nonetheless, pregnancy is one of life's richest experiences, and will be far more enjoyable if you are as relaxed as possible.

Anything that makes you feel calmer, more relaxed, in control, or able to laugh is a great tool. Whether this comes from walks with a friend, facials, or Laurel and Hardy reruns, so long as it is not bad for you or baby then it should help you enjoy the process more.

Meditation is another excellent relaxation tool, and there is convincing scientific evidence that it is highly beneficial to health and well-being. It requires only 10-15 minutes per day, and is aimed at converting negative thoughts to positive thoughts, negative energy to positive energy. The idea is that the time spent meditating is more than made up for by the increased resilience, productivity, and insight of a happy mind. It is usually taught in yoga, but can also be learned through lessons, books, tapes, etc.

Celebrate the milestones. Especially if you have had a loss, it can be difficult to relax and enjoy your pregnancy the way you would like to. Understanding how much your chances of success improve as you pass each milestone may help you feel more confident.

One large study was designed to identify milestones that would help women build confidence through pregnancy. In women who became pregnant after several consecutive miscarriages, it was found that if the embryo was confirmed alive at six weeks then there was a 78% chance of success. Once heartbeat was detected (at around seven weeks) success rate jumped to 97%. If it was confirmed alive at eight weeks, the outlook was a 98% chance of success, and at 10 weeks the chance of success was 99.4%. Based on this study it can be expected that of 1,000 women with a history of several consecutive miscarriages, 994 will have a successful pregnancy if all is confirmed well at 10 weeks.

As you reach each milestone in your own pregnancy, your confidence should increase. As discussed in *The Power of Love,* be sure to benefit from the comfort that ultrasound and other resources can give you.

Summary

So how best to enjoy pregnancy? Do whatever you can to begin your pregnancy feeling prepared and confident, and then do whatever you can to enjoy it as it unfolds.

A friend summed it up in her new year's resolution, which was just one word: Appreciate. It seems the perfect word to reflect that while we can't control everything in life, we do have a lot of control over how we react to it. Focusing on all there is to appreciate along the path to our future will make the trip a far happier one.

I wish you the greatest success, and hope that this book has helped you see more clearly the path you want to take, and to appreciate more fully the experiences along the way.

afterword

Whenever I hear that someone has suffered a miscarriage – whether a famous actress or my next door neighbor – I always wish I could do something to help, which is why I wrote *Avoiding Miscarriage*. I know how dark some of my own moments were, and anything I can do to help someone else is extremely gratifying.

If you would like to help other women in the same situation, and think this book could be of benefit to them, then please pass that information on. The more women that become aware of this book, the more miscarriages can be avoided.

I spent a year trying to find a literary agent or publisher who shared my enthusiasm for this project, all too aware that with every single minute that ticked agonizingly by, two more women miscarried and would not find this book on the shelf when they needed it. After 12 months of waiting – a million miscarriages in the US alone – I couldn't bear to delay any longer, and decided to publish the book myself. I spent my own money to get the book printed and distributed so that it could get it into the hands of the women who need it.

Thus, much as I believe this book serves a vital need, it does not have the marketing power of a major publishing house behind it. Unfortunately, this means that many women who would benefit from this book will never even know it exists.

My hope is that if the women who read this book think it is worthwhile, they will recommend it to other women, doctors, booksellers, and even the media, so that the women who need it will hear about it.

If you think other women – or the healthcare professionals who work with them – could benefit from knowing about this book, then please join in spreading the word. The following page has summary information that can be easily photocopied or cut out.

By spreading the word, each of us can help other women avoid miscarriage.

Summary information

If you would like to recommend this book, these forms may be helpful.

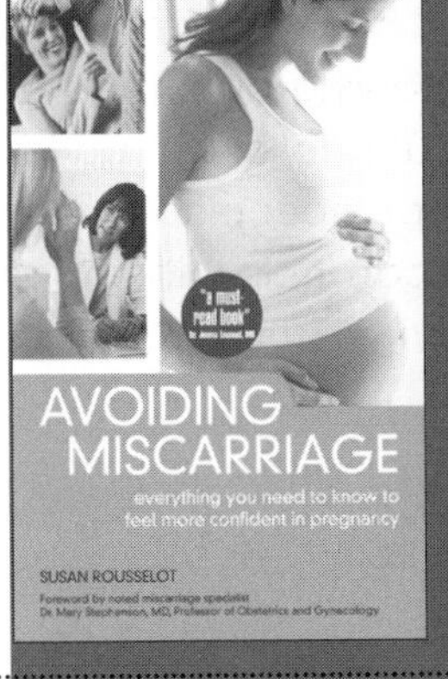

AVOIDING MISCARRIAGE
everything you need to know to
feel more confident in pregnancy

By Susan Rousselot

250 pages, paperback
ISBN: 0-9774933-1-8

For more information, or ordering:
avoidingmiscarriage.com
atlasbooks.com (also 1-800-247-6553)
or amazon.com

AVOIDING MISCARRIAGE
everything you need to know to
feel more confident in pregnancy

By Susan Rousselot

250 pages, paperback
ISBN: 0-9774933-1-8

For more information, or ordering:
avoidingmiscarriage.com
atlasbooks.com (also 1-800-247-6553)
or amazon.com

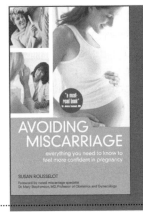

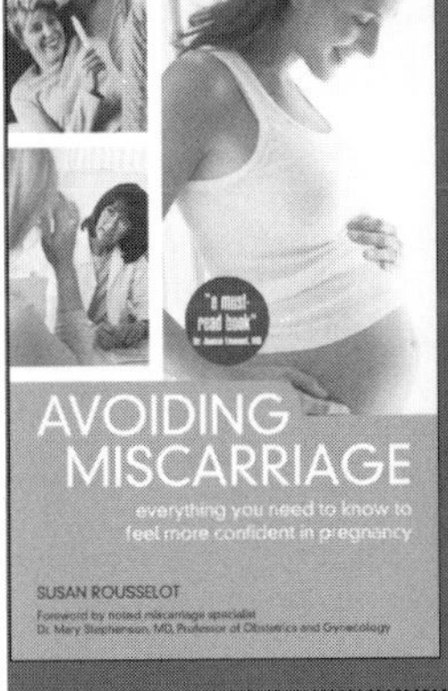

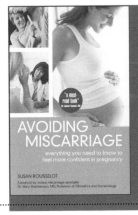

AVOIDING MISCARRIAGE
everything you need to know to
feel more confident in pregnancy

By Susan Rousselot

250 pages, paperback
ISBN: 0-9774933-1-8

For more information, or ordering:
avoidingmiscarriage.com
atlasbooks.com (also 1-800-247-6553)
or amazon.com

Nearly one in every five pregnancies ends in miscarriage.

But there's a lot you can do.

This book will help you:

- Understand how common miscarriage really is and why it happens
- Discover what might have caused any previous pregnancy loss
- Use questionnaires to assess your personal miscarriage risk profile
- Take charge of your healthcare and work effectively with your doctor
- Know what questions to ask to get the answers you need
- Identify ways to reduce your own miscarriage risk

It's time you had the information you need
to feel more confident in pregnancy.

Nearly one in every five pregnancies ends in miscarriage.

But there's a lot you can do.

This book will help you:

- Understand how common miscarriage really is and why it happens
- Discover what might have caused any previous pregnancy loss
- Use questionnaires to assess your personal miscarriage risk profile
- Take charge of your healthcare and work effectively with your doctor
- Know what questions to ask to get the answers you need
- Identify ways to reduce your own miscarriage risk

It's time you had the information you need
to feel more confident in pregnancy.

Nearly one in every five pregnancies ends in miscarriage.

But there's a lot you can do.

This book will help you:

- Understand how common miscarriage really is and why it happens
- Discover what might have caused any previous pregnancy loss
- Use questionnaires to assess your personal miscarriage risk profile
- Take charge of your healthcare and work effectively with your doctor
- Know what questions to ask to get the answers you need
- Identify ways to reduce your own miscarriage risk

It's time you had the information you need
to feel more confident in pregnancy.

glossary

Antibodies: The body's response to disease. Incorrect production of antibodies can result in the body fighting against functions that support pregnancy, or in fighting the pregnancy itself.

Antinuclear Antibodies (ANA): These antibodies are associated with excessive blood clotting which prevents adequate nourishment reaching the developing baby.

Anti-phospholipid Syndrome (APS): An immune disorder in which the mother's body produces an immune response against its own tissues or cells. APS is associated with increased blood clotting and pregnancy loss in all three trimesters.

Blastocyst: A very early stage of embryonic development, where cells form a hollow sphere with a fluid-filled cavity. The blastocyst fuses with the endometrium to form the placenta.

Blocking antibodies: These antibodies suppress the body's immune response to pregnancy, which is half comprised of foreign cells (the paternal genes), thus protecting the pregnancy from rejection.

Cervix: The narrow, neck-like end of the uterus, located at the top of the vagina.

Chromosomal Abnormalities: Errors in the division or replication of chromosomes in a developing embryo or fetus.

Chromosomes: Every human cell (except the sperm and egg cells) are comprised of 23 sets of paired chromosomes (46 chromosomes in total) which carry the many thousands of genes that make up a unique individual. Egg and sperm cells each have 23 unpaired chromosomes, which pair up at conception.

Conception: The moment when a sperm fuses with an egg.

Corpus Luteum: When a follicle matures and breaks open to release an egg into the fallopian tube, it becomes a corpus luteum which produces progesterone, instructing the body to prepare for (and later maintain) pregnancy.

DES (Diethylstilbestrol): An "anti-miscarriage" drug prescribed until the early 1970s. Women whose mothers took DES while pregnant with them have a greater risk of fertility problems, pregnancy loss, rare vaginal cancer, and reproductive organ deformation.

Dilation and Curettage (also called a "D&C"): A surgical procedure involving dilating the cervix with special instruments, and then suctioning or scraping the uterus with a curette. It is done to ensure that no "products of conception" remain in the uterus.

Ectopic Pregnancy (also called a "tubal pregnancy"): When an embryo implants outside the uterus. This is a serious medical condition requiring immediate treatment. The pregnancy cannot be saved, but the mother can be.

Embryo: The developing baby from fertilization until 10 weeks gestation (after which time it is called a "fetus").

Endometriosis: The migration of endometrial tissue to areas outside the uterus, causing pelvic pain, menstrual problems, or infertility.

Endometrium: The surface lining of the uterus, where a fertilized egg implants. This lining is shed each month as the menstrual period if conception does not occur. Then the cycle begins again with the generation of a new endometrium, which will be shed again if a viable pregnancy does not result.

Fallopian Tubes: The tubes that connect the ovaries (egg reserves) to the uterus. Fertilization actually occurs in the fallopian tubes.

Fetal Growth Restriction (also called IUGR, or "intrauterine growth retardation"): a fetus that is too small for dates.

Fetus: The developing (unborn) baby after 10 weeks gestation (prior to this it is called an "embryo.")

Follicle: Each of a woman's eggs is housed in a follicle, many thousands of which fill the ovaries. If she is not already pregnant, then each month during a woman's fertile years one of these follicles will ripen and release its egg into a fallopian tube.

Genetic Abnormalities: An error in the replication of genes in a developing embryo or fetus. Thousands of genes make up each chromosome, so a genetic abnormality is not as serious as a chromosomal one; however, a genetic abnormality could still result in miscarriage.

Heparin: A naturally occurring substance in the body, heparin reduces blood clotting and is often prescribed for women with blood clotting disorders that jeopardize pregnancy.

Hormones: Chemical substances secreted by the body to trigger effects elsewhere in the body (e.g. the hormone progesterone is secreted by the follicle after ovulation, directing the lining of the womb to soften in preparation for implantation).

Human Chorionic Gonadotropin (HCG): A hormone released by the placenta, which keeps the mother's body from initiating menstruation. Pregnancy tests detect this hormone, giving a positive result when sufficient HCG is present.

Human Leukocyte Antigen (HLA): Markers on the surface of cells that indicate a person's white blood cell type. One theory suggests that if you and your partner have too much similarity in these markers, the resultant pregnancy might trigger an immune response.

Hysterosalpingogram (HSG): An x-ray which entails the injection of a special dye into the uterus and fallopian tubes, and enables evaluation of the size, shape, and access of those structures.

Intrauterine Growth Retardation: See "Fetal Growth Restriction."

Intravenous Immunoglobulin (IVIG): IVIG is derived from blood pooled from thousands of donors that is washed and processed into a clear blend. It is thought that IVIG temporarily provides a variety of blocking antibodies that protect the pregnancy from rejection and suppress the toxic action of natural killer cells.

Karyotype: A person's unique DNA.

Karyotyping: DNA analysis to identify chromosomal profile.

Laparoscopy: A laparoscope is a long, thin, lighted viewing microscope which is used to detect and treat conditions such as endometriosis, fibroids, pelvic scar tissue, and tubal blockage.

Luteal Phase: The second half of the menstrual phase, beginning at ovulation (14 days after menstruation begins).

Luteal Phase Defect (LPD): A luteal phase (the time between ovulation and menstruation) that is out of phase: either too long or too short to enable the fertilized egg to implant properly on a healthy and receptive uterine lining.

Luteinizing Hormone (LH): The hormone responsible for stimulating an ovarian follicle to mature and release an egg.

Miscarriage: Failure of a pregnancy prior to 20 weeks gestation. The word "miscarriage" refers only to the failure of the pregnancy. The proper medical term for the expulsion of pregnancy material, which most people also call a miscarriage, is actually an "abortion." This is the term that doctors tend to use.

Mosaic: A chromosomal abnormality that does not affect 100% of the cells of an embryo or fetus. For example, if an error occurred not at conception, but at the first replication, then the embryo would be "mosaic," with 50% normal chromosomes and 50% defective.

Natural Killer (NK) Cells: Protective cells whose job it is to detect and combat foreign cells such as cancer cells. It is thought that these cells malfunction in some women, attacking the developing pregnancy as though it were a cancer.

Ovaries: The two structures containing a woman's eggs. Ovaries are formed and stocked with eggs when a woman is still in the womb herself.

Ovulation: Occurs when a follicle in the ovary releases a mature egg into the fallopian tube.

Progesterone: A hormone produced after ovulation, which signals the body to prepare for pregnancy (e.g. causing the endometrial lining to soften for implantation).

Recurrent Miscarriage: When a woman has three or more pregnancies in a row that end in miscarriage, she is labeled a "recurrent miscarrier," and her losses are considered "recurrent miscarriage."

Scan: See "Ultrasound."

Sonogram: See "Ultrasound."

Sporadic Miscarriage: Miscarriage due to random chance, rather than an underlying condition that is likely to repeat.

Stillbirth: Failure of a pregnancy after 20 weeks gestation.

Ultrasound (also called a "sonogram" or a "scan"): A procedure using high-frequency sound waves to produce a picture of the embryo or fetus, the placenta, and the reproductive structures.

Uterus (also called a "womb"): Normally about the size and shape of a small (upside-down) pear, the uterus will expand throughout pregnancy in order to accommodate the growing baby, placenta, and associated fluids.

Womb: See "uterus."

index